End of Life

A NURSE'S GUIDE TO COMPASSIONATE CARE

End of Life

A NURSE'S GUIDE TO COMPASSIONATE CARE

Lippincott Williams & Wilkins
a Wolters Kluwer business
Philadelphia · Baltimore · New York · London
Buenos Aires · Hong Kong · Sydney · Tokyo

2/07

STAFF

Executive Publisher
Judith A. Schilling McCann,
RN, MSN

Editorial Director
William J. Kelly

Clinical Director
Joan M. Robinson, RN, MSN

Senior Art Director
Arlene Putterman

Editorial Project Managers
Catherine E. Harold,
Sean Webb

Clinical Editor
Carol A. Saunderson RN, BA, BS

Editors
Toby H. Brener

Copy Editors
Beth Pitcher, Jenifer F. Walker

Designer
Susan Hopkins Rodzewich

Digital Composition Services
Diane Paluba (manager),
Joyce Rossi Biletz,
Donna S. Morris

Manufacturing
Beth J. Welsh

Editorial Assistants
Megan L. Aldinger,
Karen J. Kirk, Linda K. Ruhf

Design Assistant
Georg W. Purvis IV

Indexer
Deborah Tourtlotte

EOL010506

Library of Congress
Cataloging-in-Publication Data

End-of-life care : a nurse's guide.
    p. ; cm.
    Includes bibliographical references.
    1. Practical nursing. 2. Terminal care.
3. Palliative treatment.
    I. Lippincott Williams & Wilkins.
    [DNLM: 1. Nursing Care. 2. Terminal Care.
3. Palliative Care.
    WY 152 E557 2007]
    RT62.E53 2007
    616'.029—dc22
    ISBN 1-58255-660-1 (alk. paper)   2006002850

Contents

Contributors and consultants

Judith R. Adams, RN, BSN
Clinical Consultant
Good Health Services, Inc.
Raleigh, N.C.

Veda Alban, RN, BSN, CHPN
RN Case Manager
Hope Life Care
Ft. Myers, Fla.

Jeannette M. Anderson, RN, MSN
Nursing Consultant
JMA Nursing Consultants
Fort Worth, Tex.

Joanna E. Cain, RN, BSN, BA
President
Auctorial Pursuits, Inc.
Wilmington, N.C.

Julie A. Calvery, RN, BSN
Instructor
Carolyn McKelvey School of
    Nursing
University of Arkansas
Fort Smith

Ruth M. Carroll, APRN, BC, PhD
Faculty
Salisbury (Md.) University
    Department of Nursing

Kim Cooper, RN, MSN
Nursing Program Chair
Ivy Tech Community College of
    Indiana
Terre Haute

Lillian Craig, RN, MSN, FNP-C
Family Nurse Practitioner
Claude (Tex.) Rural Health Clinic
Instructor
Oklahoma Panhandle State
    University
Goodwell

Ariel Dyer, RN, BSN
Student, PCNP Program
Madonna University
Livonia, Mich.

Jennifer A. Emerton, RN
School Nurse
Barrington (N.H.) Middle School
Visiting Nurse
Wentworth Home Care
Dover

Cynthia L. Frozena, RN, MSN, OCN,
    CHPN
End-of-Life Consultant
Hospice Consultants of the Great
    Lakes
Manitowoc, Wis.

Cheryl Laskowski, DNS, APRN-BC
Assistant Professor
University of Vermont
Burlington

Grace G. Lewis, RN, MS, BC
Assistant Professor of Nursing
Georgia Baptist College of Nursing
    of Mercer University
Atlanta

Christina S. Melvin, APRN, MS, BC
Clinical Assistant Professor
University of Vermont
Burlington

Marg Poling, RN, BScN, PHCNP,
    MN (C)
Palliative Care Nurse Practitioner,
    Advisor
Victorian Order of Nurses,
    Thunder Bay
Ontario, Canada

Monica Narvaez Ramirez, RN, MSN
Nursing Instructor
University of the Incarnate Word
    School of Nursing & Health
    Professions
San Antonio, Tex.

Ora V. Robinson, RN, MS, PhD (C)
Director of Nursing, Vocational
    Nurse
North-West College
West Covina, Calif.

Susan Sample, RN, MSN, CRNP-BC
Program Manager, Cardiothoracic
    Surgery
Lancaster (Penn.) General Hospital

Harriet Sarnoff Schiff
Author, Lecturer
The Chelsea Forum
New York

Paula Siciliano, GNP, APRN, MS
Assistant Professor
Co-Director, Nurse Practitioner
    Program
University of Utah College of
    Nursing
Salt Lake City

Angela R. Starkweather, ACNP, PhD,
    CCRN, CNRN
Assistant Professor
Washington State University
Intercollegiate College of Nursing
Spokane

David Techner
Author, Licensed Funeral Director
Ira Kaufman Chapel
Southfield, Mich.

Allison J. Terry, RN, PhD
Director of Mental Retardation
    Community Certification
Alabama Department of Mental
    Health
Montgomery

Sheryl Thomas, RN, MSN
Nursing Instructor
Wayne County Community College
Detroit, Mich.

Robin R. Wilkerson, RN, PhD
Associate Professor of Nursing
University of Mississippi
Jackson

Sharon Wing, RN, MSN
Associate Professor
Cleveland (Ohio) State University

Dawn Zwick, RN, APRN-BC, MSN
Instructor
Kent (Ohio) State University

PART ONE

Understanding end-of-life care

1

Concepts of palliative care

Depending on the circumstances and the setting in which your patient dies, end-of-life care may last moments or months. It may involve complex drug regimens and near constant symptomatic care, or it may involve only honest, compassionate conversations with family members. Either way, you have acted to ease a patient's transition from life to death.

Most Americans don't die rapidly of a sudden illness. Instead, we're more likely to be disabled for months or years by heart disease, emphysema, cancer, or another serious long-term illness. We have episodes of recurring complications, and we finally die "suddenly" as a result of an illness that has likely been present for years.

In the next 30 years, the number of older Americans will continue to grow at an increasing rate. In 2000, 4.2 million Americans were age 85 or older. By 2030, the baby-boom cohort of the 1950s will begin to hit age 85 and face the prospect of substantial disability. At that time, nearly 9 million Americans will be older than age 85 and will have some form of disease process that may lead to a discussion of end-of-life issues.

Your ability to incorporate the skills and the mindset of palliative care at the proper moment can help dying patients and their families attain a physically and spiritually peaceful death.

Defining palliative care

The notion of palliative care has existed for little more than a single generation. (See *History of end-of-life care*.) Even so, its tenets and benefits are becoming widely known. Many agencies and organizations have issued definitions for palliative care. They all have certain points in common. In general, palliative care seeks to prevent and relieve suffering and to enhance the patient's comfort and quality of life. It may be delivered alongside curative medical care, or it may be delivered alone as end-of-life care, seeking neither to delay nor hasten the patient's death.

Especially in an end-of-life setting, palliative care seeks to ease all aspects of suffering, not just the physical ravages of disease or disability. For a dying patient, palliative care addresses psychological, spiritual, and practical issues in addition to those—such as pain or nausea—caused directly by a disease.

History of end-of-life care

1967 Dame Cicely Saunders founds the first modern hospice— St. Christopher's—in London and introduces the concept in the U.S. while lecturing at Yale.

1969 Dr. Elisabeth Kübler-Ross publishes *On Death and Dying,* starting a grassroots movement in the U.S.

1978 The first U.S. hospice is founded in New Haven, Connecticut.

1978 National Hospice Organization (NHO) is founded.

1980 Congress establishes a 2-year demonstration program in 27 hospices to test improved health care for terminally ill patients.

1982 Congress passes the Medicare Hospice Benefit under Medicare Part A.

1987 Hospice Nurses Association (HNA) is formed.

1990 World Health Organization defines hospice and palliative care to set international standards.

1990 Congress passes the Patient Self-Determination Act, giving patients the right to advance directives and choices in their medical care.

1994 First nurses are certified as hospice specialists through the National Board for Certification of Hospice Nurses.

1997 HNA becomes the Hospice and Palliative Nurses Association.

1999 Certification of Hospice and Palliative Nurses begins.

2000 NHO becomes the National Hospice and Palliative Care Organization.

Typically, palliative care is provided by an interdisciplinary team on which a nurse plays a pivotal, personal role. Ideally, the nurse in collaboration with the palliative care team can address each of the patient's and family's needs. The patient and family are viewed as a single unit of care. Great emphasis is placed on meeting the patient's needs and wishes, always in the context of the family as a unit.

When palliative care succeeds, the patient dies what some call a "good" death, free from avoidable distress and suffering, in keeping with his and his family's wishes, and according to accepted clinical and ethical standards.

Philosophy of palliative care

In 1997, a task force sponsored by the Robert Wood Johnson Foundation developed this philosophy of hospice and palliative care.

■ Palliative care provides support and care for persons facing life-threatening illnesses across settings.

■ Palliative care is based on the understanding that dying is a part of the normal life cycle.

■ The process of dying is a profound individual experience.

■ Care is focused on enhancing the quality of remaining life by integrating physical, psychological, social, and spiritual aspects of care.

■ Use of an interdisciplinary team is the key to addressing the many needs of the dying and their families. (See *Elements of palliative care.*)

■ Interventions affirm life and neither hasten nor postpone death.

■ Through appropriate care and the promotion of a caring community, patients and families may be free to realize a degree of satisfaction and closure in preparing for death.

The nurse's role

Expert nursing care is essential in end-of-life situations. (See *Standards of hospice and palliative nursing care,* page 6.) Of all the health care providers involved in end-of-life care, it's the nurse who spends the most time with the patient and family. The nurse provides the type of care that allows patients and families to grow in the dying experience. Through expert nursing care, patients and families may experience the final phase of life as one that is healing, growth producing, even transformative.

Nurses have a wonderful opportunity to influence not only individual patients and families but also policy development in end-of-life care. Clinically, nurses are pivotal in providing symptom management. On a community and national level, nurses can lobby for progressive means to provide effective end-of-life care. This might include an expanded Hospice Medicare Benefit, more community resources for families unable to care for a terminally patient at home, and fundraising to support end-of-life care and education.

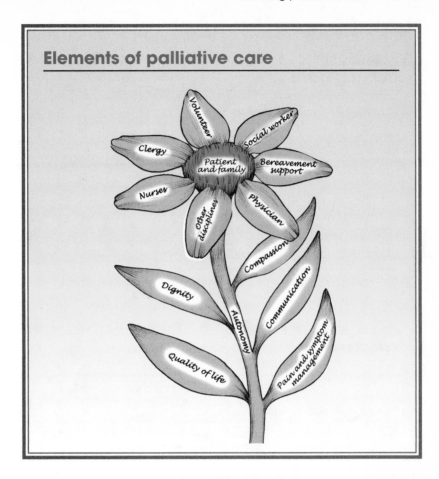

Elements of palliative care

Terminally ill patients and their families deserve expert nursing care. By participating in the reality of end-of-life conditions, nurses accept the feelings of the individual. Caring for people in this phase of life acknowledges their deepest pain, legitimizes their experience, and gives them a feeling of personal integrity, wholeness, and value. As nurses discuss dying and death, they must do so in the context of hope, meaning, and continued growth and autonomy. In doing so, nurses continuously educate patients, families and others that death is a natural part of life.

Nurses are instrumental in ensuring that patients at the end of life are not abandoned. Nurses remain at the bedside, in the home, or in the nursing home. Nurses' professional and personal ethics insist on acknowledging and honoring the patient's wishes. Patients expect nurses to be available to them and, in doing so, nurses commit to experience the process with the patient. A core nursing function is to bear witness and be present with our patients as they move through the dying process and ultimately to help them find meaning in the experience. What is demanded of nurses is to pro-

Standards of hospice and palliative nursing care

Standard	Action
Assessment	Collect basic patient and family data.
Diagnosis	Analyze the assessment data and determine diagnoses using an accepted framework that supports hospice and palliative nursing knowledge.
Outcome identification	Identify expected outcomes relevant to the patient and family, in partnership with the interdisciplinary team.
Planning	Develop a plan of care—negotiated among patient, family, and interdisciplinary team—that includes interventions and treatments to attain expected outcomes.
Implementation	Implement the interventions identified in the plan of care.
Evaluation	Evaluate the patient's and family's progress in attaining expected outcomes.

From *Scope and Standards of Hospice and Palliative Nursing Practice,* Hospice and Palliative Nurses Association and American Nurses Association, 2002.

vide expert assessment, critical thinking, and symptom management with compassion and respect for the patient and his family.

Key nursing interventions

Besides the nursing interventions needed to provide excellent clinical care, certain interventions are particularly helpful during end-of-life care. They include presence, compassion, touch, recognition of the patient's autonomy, honesty, expert communication skills, and assisting with transcendence.

Presence
Presence is a core nursing intervention that can be described as a "gift of self" in which you are available and open to the situation. You may show your presence through verbal communication, valuing what the patient

says, accepting the patient's meanings for things, connecting, fostering an inner understanding or intuition, and remembering or reflecting.

Compassion
Compassion is another fundamental element in nursing care. Without human compassion for the dying, growth and healing are unlikely to occur. It's your ability to be totally and compassionately with the patient and family that allows the most positive experience for patient and family, and for you.

Touch
Through touch, you and the patient are linked, and you can offer unconditional acceptance. Touch is a powerful therapeutic intervention. For people who are dying, touch can be both a healing and a life-affirming act whereby you communicate genuine caring and compassion. Furthermore, touch can convey to a patient that he is safe to freely express any concerns or needs. This type of connectedness with patients helps to mitigate suffering.

Recognition of autonomy
Self-rule is typically considered to be a fundamental element of hospice care. This element especially comes into play as advance directives are considered. Although he may collaborate with family, significant others, and the palliative care team, the patient has the right to make all end-of-life decisions.

Honesty
Often, it's the nurse who ultimately interprets the real implications of the diagnosis and prognosis given to the patient and family by the physician. Patients expect nurses to be honest. In these situations, the patient and family need and deserve honesty regarding the day-to-day effects of the medical findings and what the patient may expect in the days ahead. Through compassionate honesty, you can build trust with the patient and family.

Expert communication
Inherent in these interventions is the need for expert communication skills. At any given moment, it will be up to you to assess the patient and family, to devise a plan to best comfort them, and to communicate clearly and supportively throughout.

Assisting in transcendence
Literally, transcendence means to triumph over something. In end-of-life care, transcendence refers to a patient developing a sense of meaning and

peace that keeps his suffering and death from being meaningless. At the highest level of nursing care, you can provide emotional support that lets a patient experience self-transcendence and a sort of triumph in death.

For this to occur, you must become a willing partner in the patient's journey to death. He will experience intense pain, abandonment, and fear of living and dying in an effort to construct meaning from seemingly meaningless experiences—and you'll experience some portion of these feelings as well. The development of meaning is a dynamic process that requires engaged listening, authentic responsiveness, mutual disclosure, and negotiation. It's among the highest goals of palliative care.

Defining hospice care

Hospice is an organized, legally defined concept in which end-of-life care is delivered. Although end-of-life care can take place in almost any setting and for widely varying lengths of time, many people who know they will die choose to receive end-of-life care through hospice services.

Philosophy of hospice care

The philosophy of hospice care aligns closely with that of palliative care. For example:

■ It exists for persons in the last phases of incurable disease to help them live as fully and as comfortably as possible.

■ It recognizes dying as a part of the normal process of living.

■ It focuses on enhancing the quality of remaining life.

■ It affirms life and neither hastens nor postpones death.

■ It exists in the hope and belief that patients and families may attain a degree of satisfaction in preparation for death.

■ It recognizes that human growth and development can be a lifelong process.

■ It seeks to preserve and promote the potential for growth in patients and families during the last phase of life.

■ It offers palliative care for all patients and their families without regard to age, gender, nationality, race, creed, sexual orientation, disability, diagnosis, and ability to pay.

Key concepts in hospice care

Certain concepts are key to the provision of hospice services and are outlined here.

Unit of care

The patient and family (as defined by the patient) are considered a single unit of care. Some families come to hospice with many unresolved issues; others don't. Part of the care provided by the team is to help patients and families address these issues. This may include developing a living will and durable power of attorney for both financial and health care needs, or it may include resolving longstanding family disputes or a myriad of other issues.

Interdisciplinary team

An interdisciplinary team is used to address the physical, social, emotional, and spiritual needs of the patient and family. The interdisciplinary team includes physicians, nurses, social workers, volunteer coordinators, clergy, bereavement coordinators, and any other discipline needed to provide holistic care (a physical therapist or speech therapist, for example).

The purpose of the team is to deliver well-coordinated interdisciplinary care. (See *Standards of performance in hospice and palliative nursing,* page 10.) Typically, the team discusses each patient and family in a weekly meeting and updates the care plan accordingly. The team closely monitors disease progression, keeping in mind that additional services may need to be added.

Medical treatment

Hospice provides treatment for pain and other distressing symptoms of terminal illness but doesn't seek to cure disease, prolong life, or hasten death. Compared to patients who don't select hospice for end-of-life care, those who do choose hospice tend to receive more regular pain management, particularly with morphine derivatives, and significant improvements in physical and emotional symptoms. Many symptoms can be addressed at once in hospice care, including pain, dyspnea, nausea, vomiting, restlessness, agitation, fear, confusion, anxiety, depression, and loneliness.

Holistic care

Based on the wishes of patient and family, the interdisciplinary team develops a plan of care to provide coordinated, supportive services such as home care, pain management, and limited inpatient services. Typically, when a patient enters hospice, the nurse develops a plan of care. The interdisciplinary team then reviews the plan of care weekly and makes adjustments accordingly.

The shift from curative to hospice care allows the patient to be treated in a holistic manner that includes physical, emotional, social, economic, and spiritual needs; the patient's response to illness; and the effect of the illness on the patient's ability to meet his own needs.

Standards of performance in hospice and palliative nursing

Standard	Action
Quality of care	Systematically evaluate the quality and effectiveness of hospice and palliative nursing practice.
Performance appraisal	Evaluate your own nursing practice in relation to professional practice standards and relevant statutes and regulations.
Education	Acquire and maintain current knowledge and competency in hospice and palliative care nursing.
Collegiality	Interact with and contribute to the professional development of peers and other health care providers as colleagues.
Ethics	Show moral discernment, critical reasoning, and discriminating judgment in integrating ethics into hospice and palliative nursing during all interactions with the patient, family, organization, and community.
Collaboration	Collaborate with patient, family, members of the interdisciplinary team, and other health care providers in providing patient and family care.
Research	Use research findings in practice.
Use of resources	Consider factors related to safety, effectiveness, and cost in planning and delivering patient and family care.

From *Scope and Standards of Hospice and Palliative Nursing Practice*, Hospice and Palliative Nurses Association and the American Nurses Association, 2002.

Volunteer support

Hospice care actively engages the community by using volunteer support to deliver hospice services. Volunteers are trained to deal with the ill and dying. Often, the training program has as many as 30 hours of education in all aspects of hospice care. After completing the training program, the volunteer can be assigned a patient and family by the hospice agency's volunteer coordinator.

The activities that a volunteer can do vary widely. They may involve staying with the patient so the family can rest, do errands, or attend appointments. They also may include such activities as bringing food to the patient, reading to the patient, and writing letters for the patient.

Hospice setting

The patient's primary residence is the primary site of hospice care. In other words, hospice is not setting-specific. Originally, much of hospice care was delivered in the home. Today, hospice care is delivered in a variety of places that include the home, nursing or residential facilities, homes for the terminally ill, or any other site where the patient is living.

Bereavement support

Hospice emphasizes comfort, dignity, and quality of life, with the focus on spiritual and existential issues throughout dying, death, and bereavement. Hospices have bereavement support available to all surviving family members. Clergy are an integral part of the interdisciplinary team and are available during the dying process and after the patient's death. Many hospices offer bereavement support groups as well.

Control

In hospice, the patient and family are in the driver's seat. They have the right to choose where end-of-life care is delivered and specify the details of the patient's dying process. For instance, they decide whether the patient will eat or drink, which foods and liquids will be consumed, and which drugs will be taken. At some point, the patient may choose to stop eating and drinking. Drugs may be stopped either by choice or the patient's inability to swallow. Many decisions can and should be made using advance directives. These include a living will, durable power of attorney for health care, and organ donation card. Throughout end-of-life care, the hospice physician and nurse work to keep the patient informed about the progress of his condition and to solicit his wishes.

Medicare and hospice

In 1982, Congress created the Medicare Hospice Benefit (MHB) under Medicare Part A. This benefit was the first formal recognition that dying people have unique needs, and it clearly stated that Congress acknowledged those needs. The benefit established an all-inclusive package of services for patients with a life expectancy of 6 months or less.

This program provides services mainly in patients' homes, with home health agencies providing care. (See *Medicare hospice services*, page 12.) Services are designed to provide for the physical, psychosocial, spiritual, and financial needs of the patient and family—as defined by the patient. MHB services that are covered under Medicare Part A include:
- physician and nursing care

Medicare hospice services

Four types of services are included under the Medicare hospice program.

Type of service	Characteristics
Routine home care	■ Care typically provided in patient's home. ■ Hospice staff provides full scope of services.
Continuous home care	■ More intensive care in the home. ■ Patient needs skilled nursing care for at least 8 hours of the 24-hour day. ■ Typically used for acute symptom management to prevent the need for hospitalization.
Respite inpatient care	■ Patient moves to an inpatient facility to give caregivers respite from physical and emotional stresses of end-of-life care. ■ Maximum of 5 days per admission for respite.
General inpatient care	■ Patient is admitted to an inpatient facility for acute problems that need medical and nursing management. ■ Days may be limited.

■ home health aide and homemaker services
■ physical, occupational, and speech therapy
■ social work and counseling services
■ chaplin services
■ volunteer support (such as help with shopping, companionship, respite for the family)
■ bereavement counseling
■ medical equipment and supplies
■ drugs related to the disease
■ inpatient care for up to 5 days at a time in a Medicare-approved facility for symptom management, respite for caregivers, or both.

Medicaid and hospice

Medicaid is a program for the poor, the disabled, and children. The Medicaid Hospice Benefit is patterned after the version adopted by Medicare, although states have some flexibility in services covered because Medicaid is a combination of federal and state dollars. Medicaid is the payer of last choice, after all other insurers, including Medicare, have been billed.

Length of stay

One of the main keys to success for patients in hospice is a long enough length of stay. Hospice experts note that the longer a person receives hospice care, the better the outcome for symptom management and personal and family coping.

Clearly, it can be difficult to accurately predict the length of a patient's remaining life, particularly if the patient has Alzheimer's disease, end-stage cardiac disease, or a neurologic disorder. Late referrals may occur for other reasons as well, mainly confusion about when the referral is most appropriate.

It's imperative for the referral to occur in time for adequate services to be delivered. Adequate pain control is possible in most situations, but it takes time to adjust the drugs for maximum effect. Currently, the median length of survival in hospice is about 20 days. About one-third of patients die within 7 days of their referral.

As the public and professional mindset changes from death as a medical failure to death as a natural part of life, referrals will likely be made earlier. That way, the hospice team can better address all aspects of patient care, including those that offer the patient and family a more autonomous process and one filled with more meaning.

2 Essential communication skills

When a patient is dying, compassionate communication becomes a clinical skill as important as assessment, drug administration, and physical intervention. The fact is that nurses are in the best position to help dying patients communicate about their wishes, help families understand the course of the patient's transition, ease conflicts and difficulties that are sure to arise (see *Allowing acceptance*), and facilitate interactions with physicians and other members of the palliative care team.

When communicating with a patient and family members, always take care to convert medical language into lay language, not only to increase the patient's and family's understanding but also to better invite them into the conversation. Also, keep in mind that many families have varying educational levels, reading abilities, and language preferences. To communicate effectively with patients and their families, make sure you're communicating with cultural sensitivity, building rapport, using empathy, participating as needed in important end-of-life decisions, and continuously assessing yourself and your effectiveness.

Cultural sensitivity

The percentage of families ethnically and culturally different from the prevailing European model continues to climb. In the United States Census of 2000, respondents identified themselves this way:

- 65% white
- 13% black
- 13% Hispanic

EXPERT INSIGHTS

Allowing acceptance

A physician I work with routinely orders psychiatric consults for termi-
nally ill patients who ask her to stop aggressive treatment. Do you
think that's warranted? — S.S., Ohio

No. I think it's usually an indication that the physician is uncomfortable
caring for a patient at the end of life. Some physicians also want to
verify and document a patient's competence for legal reasons.

Recently I got a referral to see a patient terminally ill with lung cancer and liver metastasis. His physician wanted me to talk with him
about going to rehab so he could get strong enough to tolerate more
chemotherapy.

I found my patient lying in bed staring up at the ceiling. I introduced myself as a clinical specialist who works exclusively with people
who are seriously ill. I then asked if he wanted to talk about how things
were going.

He simply said, "I'm fine."

I went on to say that I was terribly sorry that the cancer had gotten
away from us and that I wondered what he wanted now.

"I just want to go home."

"Home to heaven or home to your house, Mr. North?"

"Both."

I mentioned that his chart said he hadn't eaten for many days,
and I asked if he wanted to try an appetite stimulant.

"No. I'm fine."

I asked if he had any questions or concerns he wanted to discuss,
and he just shook his head no. But as I got to the door he said, "Joy,
I've got no reason to lie to you. I'm done, and I'm fine."

I reminded him that he could ask for me if he wanted to talk, and
then I went to write my note in his chart.

The next day, Mr. North's excellent nurse paged me. "You'll never
believe what Dr. Sutherland did!" she exclaimed. "He ordered a psych
consult for Mr. North to find out why he won't eat!"

"Mr. North doesn't need a psych consult. He's not eating because
he's lost his appetite and he's ready to die," I said emphatically.

The psychiatrist's consultation was brief and to the point. Her note
simply said that the patient wasn't suicidal and that he was well-
adjusted and accepted his terminal condition.

(continued)

Allowing acceptance *(continued)*

I believe that, at certain times, some terminally ill patients can benefit from psychiatry and antidepressant treatment. But it's a mistake to routinely order consults for patients just because they recognize and accept their condition.

This approach is a glaring reminder of how poorly some health care providers deal with death and dying. Sorrow over leaving the planet isn't an abnormal reaction that requires analysis. Most dying patients find great comfort in just being able to share their feelings with someone who's caring and empathetic.

By the way, Mr. North went home the next day with a hospice referral.

— *JOY UFEMA, RN, MS*

- 4.5% Asian–Pacific islander
- 1.5% American Indian–Alaskan native
- 2.5% bi-ethnic.

All told, at least one-third of the patients and families you care for will be part of an ethnic or cultural minority. To establish good communication, it's increasingly important to assess differences in values, priorities, customs, and goals among a culturally diverse population.

For instance, some cultures may view discussing serious illness or bad news harmful to the patient, as well as being disrespectful or impolite. Thus, family members may communicate from the perspective of protecting their loved one. Some cultures believe that open discussion of illness may provoke depression or anxiety. Others believe that discussing an illness may eliminate hope or that speaking out loud about the possibility of death could make it come true.

For example, a Navajo may believe that negative words and thoughts about health will become a reality. Because you spoke it, so it will be. The Navajo place a prominent value on positive thinking and speaking, a value that can make it difficult to openly discuss advance directives or end-of-life care. Chinese patients tend not to discuss advance directives either because of a similar belief that what one says will become a self-fulfilling prophecy. Chinese patients also hold their elderly in high esteem and don't want them to be upset by bad news. In Asian cultures, it's perceived as cruel to inform a patient of a cancer diagnosis.

Another communication problem may arise if the physician's cultural background reduces the motivation to discuss end-of-life issues, which might give patients a sense of false hope. Differing views on end-of-life issues by both patients and health care professionals may translate into a lower likelihood of advance directives. One study found that 40% of older white patients had completed advance directives compared to only 16% of older black patients.

In summary, when communicating about end-of-life issues, many cultural variables come into play, including respect, causing harm, provoking anxiety or depression, and self-fulfilling prophecy. Use therapeutic listening to let the patient and family voice their concerns. And be attentive to issues of acceptance, tying up loose ends, voicing anger, and preparing for death.

Rapport

No matter what their cultural heritage, before you can communicate effectively with a patient or family, you'll need to develop rapport with them. Having rapport means that you can communicate with harmony, affinity, and cooperation. Start building rapport at your very first meeting. (See *Fostering rapport.*)

Before you say a word, your body posture and your gestures will begin the process of building or blocking rapport. At your first contact with a patient, you'll need to present a calm demeanor. Stay aware of any cultural

Fostering rapport

Here are some quick tips to help you build rapport with patients and family members.

- Use open body language and gestures.
- Focus on the person who is speaking.
- Use silence to show concern and understanding.
- Eliminate distractions, both environmental and mental.
- Be culturally aware.
- Ask open-ended questions.
- Offer empathy rather than sympathy.

To say or not to say

When working with dying patients and their families, you may find it difficult to know what to say to comfort them. Here are some examples of what to say — and what not to say.

What to say
- What do you need me to do for you?
- Is there anyone I can call for you?
- I'm here to listen.
- No need to rush. Take your time.
- It's okay to cry. Let me get you a tissue.
- Would you like to be left alone?
- Would you like to share some memories?

What not to say
- She's in a better place now.
- He lived a full life.
- She's out of her pain.
- It'll be alright.
- Don't cry.
- Be strong.
- He'd want you to get on with your life.

variables that could disrupt your ability to build rapport. For example, some cultures find direct eye contact disrespectful. Cultural competence is essential to knowing what a patient may find disrespectful.

Another key to developing rapport is listening closely, being fully present, and being aware of the patient's feelings without losing the theme of the conversation. If the culture permits, sit at eye level. Focus on the person speaking. Use silence as well as words to show your willingness to be present. Encourage honest sharing of feelings, exude a demeanor of patience, and use all available resources. Listen to the message and not just the words. Try to identify whether your patient is communicating physical, emotional, or spiritual messages. Understanding the broad category of your patient's concern can help you ask more pertinent follow-up questions.

Also, eliminate distractions, both environmental and mental. Resist thinking about other tasks or other patients. Even if you're not feeling well or you have some other kind of discomfort, do your best to move your struggle to a back burner and be present with your dying patient and his family. Doing so will foster a supportive environment.

Maintaining communication, a good rapport, and a supportive environment also means giving up any judgments you have about the patient. Try to understand not just the disease process but the person's perceptions of the disease or end-of-life issues. Don't view the patient as a case, a disease, or a group of symptoms.

Focus on the patient holistically. Consider physical, mental, emotional, and spiritual aspects. Weigh the overall daily challenges of caring for the patient. Promote environmental comfort—which includes the family as an environment of comfort—and remember your role as advocate for your patient.

Also, take steps to avoid saying things to a dying patient or his family that won't be helpful. (See *To say or not to say*.) Certain statements, though well-meaning, will only discount their feelings of loss. Things will not be okay. Someone may be losing a lifelong companion, a child, and financial stability in addition to companionship. Even those in abusive relationships may have deep feelings of loss. Make sure to communicate in a way that opens the door for patients and families to talk about their feelings.

Empathy

Remember that empathy—rather than sympathy or pity—lets you see the problem from the patient's point of view without taking on the burden of the patient's situation. (See *Communicating with empathy*, page 20.) Your ability to understand your patient's feelings without becoming mired in them yourself is essential. Becoming enmeshed in the patient's feelings may cause physical or psychological distress, making you less effective as a therapeutic listener.

Listen actively to your patient's concerns. When responding, use empathetic statements. Also, ask open-ended questions, such as:

- What do you hope for as you live with this condition?
- What do you fear?
- If you were to die soon, what would be left undone in your life?
- How are things going for you and your family?

Empathetic communication lets the patient voice his concerns and needs. It lets him feel heard. It also shows that you're concerned about the patient and not just about finishing a task.

COMFORT & CARE

Communicating with empathy

When caring for a terminally ill patient, an empathetic rather than a sympathetic approach will open more doors to honest communication, make you better able to determine your patient's needs and goals, and reduce your risk of exhaustion and burnout. Here's how to tell the difference between empathy and sympathy.

Empathy
When you communicate with empathy, you gain an emotional appreciation of another person's feelings. You strive to understand that person's experience from inside his unique frame of reference. Examples of empathetic questions and statements include:
- Can you tell me more about that?
- Let me see if I understand you correctly.
- It sounds like that makes you feel . . .

Sympathy
When you communicate with sympathy, you share the person's suffering, taking it onto and into yourself and feeling what the patient feels. By doing so, you become less able to help and more at risk of burnout and exhaustion. Examples of sympathetic questions and statements include:
- I feel your pain.
- I know how you feel.
- I'm so sorry for you.

End-of-life decisions

Communicating about the nuts and bolts of end-of-life decisions may seem outside the realm of nursing, but it isn't when you're caring for a dying patient and his family. To advocate effectively for your patient, you may need to get involved in a myriad of decisions that may, at first, seem surprising.

For example, a major end-of-life decision is whether or not to pay bills. Some patients won't want to. For others, continuing to participate in activities of daily living—through paying bills, in this case—can help maintain a sense of control over what remains of their life. For still others, paying one's debts may reflect spiritual or religious convictions.

Another end-of-life decision involves which family members, friends, colleagues, and acquaintances to tell, what to tell them, how to tell them, and when to tell them. Some patients may not wish to disclose that they're dying, even to loved ones.

Making funeral arrangements is another major task. Some patients may want to plan their own funeral and do all the calling, ordering the flowers, arranging the caterer, and so on. Performing or supervising these tasks can help maintain the patient's sense of control, dignity, and empowerment. It also can reduce the risk of family disputes over what the patient might have wanted, such as the type of flowers, the wording of the obituary, which picture to display, whether to remove jewelry, and what clothing the patient will wear.

End-of-life decisions commonly include which treatments to elect, which to decline, and when. For example, cancer patients may need to decide between traditional and alternative treatments, to have chemotherapy or not, to have radiation therapy or not. When talking with the patient about treatments, be honest. Discuss the adverse effects (such as hair loss with chemotherapy) and the treatments used to alleviate symptoms. In cases like this, don't be surprised if your patient knows more than you do about his disease process and related alternative therapies.

If the patient is a single parent, the major end-of-life decision may involve who will be designated to care for the children. If the patient has a same-sex partner, the major end-of-life decision may involve making sure that worldly possessions pass peacefully to that person. Of course, this decision also may arise if the patient has an opposite-sex partner but isn't married.

No matter what the patient's personal or family situation, you must be sensitive to each patient's needs and requests without judgment or bias. This is the only way you can deliver the best care, compassionately. One of the most grueling decisions may involve whether or not to have a "do not resuscitate" (DNR) order. Take a moment to ask yourself, "How do I feel about DNR orders?" How do your religious or spiritual beliefs influence your answer? How do these feelings alter the care you're comfortable providing? Would you request a change in patient assignments?

Another end-of-life decision is about organ donation. Patients may be in conflict, depending upon their disease process and spirituality, about whether their organs could be of use to anyone.

When communicating with the patient or family members, reduce your language to the eloquence of simplicity. Be matter-of-fact and empathetic. Give accurate information. Listen actively and, if appropriate, use gentle touch to show your care and concern.

Self-assessment

To communicate compassionately and well with dying patients and their families, you must continually assess your strengths and weaknesses in this area. Ask yourself questions like these:

■ How do I feel about end-of-life issues?

■ How do I feel about discussing spirituality?

■ How do I feel about discussing spirituality when the patient's spiritual views conflict with mine?

■ How do I handle the grieving process?

■ Have I had personal experiences with the grieving process that could hinder my effectiveness?

■ Do I have an ethical dilemma that could interfere with my ability to communicate with patients and families about end-of-life issues?

■ Do I harbor any bias toward any race, cultural or ethnic group, lifestyle, or disease that could interfere with my care and compassion?

■ Do I use avoidance as a coping mechanism?

■ Do I forgive myself for my human inadequacies?

■ Do I internalize negative behavior from patients?

If you tend to avoid emotional situations, you may not let yourself get involved enough in the deeply emotional process of end-of-life care. If, on the other hand, you tend to rescue others from painful situations or decisions, you may get overly involved in the family's dynamics. Knowing and accepting yourself will help you stay appropriately involved and will guide you in communicating clearly and compassionately with patients and their families.

Ethical considerations

When caring for dying patients, you'll almost certainly encounter ethical challenges as varied as the patients themselves. However, certain topics tend to arise over and over. Some of the most common areas of ethical concern involve when and how to shift from curative to palliative care, establishing trust with the patient and family, refocusing hope for the patient and family, providing appropriate information, maintaining confidentiality and privacy, relieving the patient's pain, and withdrawing treatment.

Entering end-of-life care

At some point during a failing treatment process, the focus begins to shift from cure to palliation, and end-of-life care begins. The decision to enter hospice or simply to begin gradually stopping aggressive treatments rests first and foremost with the patient. The patient is the only one who knows when it's time to stop seeking aggressive or curative treatments and instead to seek comfort measures and support for quality of life throughout the dying process.

Of course, it's important for the family—however the patient defines that term—to be involved in deciding when the time is most appropriate to move from cure to care. But ultimately, the final decision rests exclusively with the patient. Establishing and protecting this right for the patient and his family is your ethical responsibility, allowing the patient to maintain a sense of control over his future and his autonomy as an adult.

Establishing trust and refocusing hope

In end-of-life care, as much as in any arena of nursing, mutual trust forms the foundation of a therapeutic nurse-patient relationship. The patient must be able to trust that you are both competent and knowledgeable, a capable and reliable practitioner. In return, you must be able to trust that the patient is providing accurate information and expressing thoughts and feelings to the best of his ability. This is the only way you can confidently plan and provide care that meets the patient's physical, emotional, spiritual, and cultural needs. When trust is breached on either side of the relationship, your ability to help the patient achieve his goals is threatened.

Before making the decision to begin end-of-life care, the patient and his family may have hoped for cure, for recovery, for life to continue as it was before the patient became seriously ill. Once the patient decides to change his treatment focus, he takes the first step toward his individualized dying process. To navigate this process, he and his family must recognize the futility of their earlier hopes, a recognition that can be even more devastating if it leads to hopelessness.

Hope is an intangible quality that lets us overlook a present discomfort in order to achieve a desired goal. One of your most important roles — both clinical and ethical — at this time is to help the patient and family maintain a sense of hope by refocusing on attainable goals. (See *Transforming the meaning of hope.*)

This task isn't easy, and you may struggle with the awkward balance between truthfulness and hopefulness. In fact, years ago, it was common for physicians to withhold a diagnosis of terminal disease in an effort to keep the patient from sinking into hopelessness. Some even created an elaborate pretense to avoid discussing the inevitability of the patient's death, instead choosing to manipulate conversations in the hope that the patient would discover the truth of his diagnosis for himself without being told by others. Although remnants of this kind of thinking remain, especially among physicians uncomfortable discussing death, experts in death and dying agree that this approach removes the patient's autonomy and opportunity to complete crucial goals before he dies.

Naturally, you never want to dispense information in a callous or insensitive way, even if what you say is technically true. For example, in even the bleakest situation, never say that nothing more can be done for the patient. (See *Power of suggestion*, page 26.) Be honest with the patient about the symptoms he likely will experience and the methods that can be used to manage those symptoms. Explain that his care team will do everything possible to ease his transition. And help the patient refocus his hope.

Hope for a patient approaching the end of life can be maintained through the idea of transcending self. This can occur as the patient reaches out to

COMFORT & CARE

Transforming the meaning of hope

When a patient and his family must relinquish their hope for recovery, you can help refocus their hope to other important, attainable goals, such as these:
- Hope for a comfortable death without pain or discomfort
- Hope for the patient to reaffirm — or discover for the first time — the value of his life
- Hope for the resolution of unresolved issues
- Hope for the patient's affirmation or discovery of comforting spiritual beliefs
- Hope for quality of life
- Hope for the patient's ability to accomplish his wishes during his final days

others, accepts help, experiences pleasure from his surroundings, and reminisces about his life. Meaning can be found through creation of a legacy, letting go of meaningless activities, and living in the moment. The end of life can be seen as a time of reflection, achievement, and continued opportunity. With this view, it's clear that failure to disclose important information at appropriate times and with the appropriate sensitivity may limit or remove the patient's opportunities for growth and satisfaction with his life.

In addition, address the patient's specific needs. Help him understand and embrace the things for which he can hope, including that he'll have:
- care throughout the dying process — that he won't be abandoned
- culturally respectful care
- as much autonomy and personal control as possible
- permission and encouragement to reflect on the implications of his diagnosis and prognosis; to identify and explore his thoughts, feelings, and needs; to tell his story often and in detail; to reaffirm his identify and the value of his life; to reflect on his life and to grieve current and past losses
- time with family and friends
- time to address unfinished personal business, to complete financial responsibilities, and to plan for the distribution of his assets
- help in discussing, developing, and finalizing the documents that pertain to end-of-life decision-making
- accurate, timely, reliable information at a level of detail tailored to his wishes

EXPERT INSIGHTS

Power of suggestion

Last week I overheard an oncology nurse tell a patient receiving chemotherapy that his type of cancer has no cure. The patient, who'd been responding well to treatment, told me later that although he knew his prognosis was poor, her comments made him wonder, What's the point? Now he's thinking about stopping chemotherapy.

When I spoke to the nurse about how her remarks had affected the patient, she said she was doing him a favor by telling him the truth. According to her, "It's not right to give patients false hope."
What do you think? — C.W., Alberta

Not only is giving a prognosis way outside a nurse's scope of practice, a statement like hers is insensitive and unethical.

Thirty-two years ago I sat in a lecture hall and heard Elisabeth Kübler-Ross tell us never to take away a patient's hope. Hope is always available, no matter how poor the prognosis. It's a lesson I've never forgotten.

Regardless of prognosis, a nurse's attitude can influence a patient's survival and quality of life. Consider this study: Nurses gave analgesics to two groups of patients. With one group, they interacted minimally. With the other group, they spoke softly, exuded caring and empathy, and reassured patients that the drug would ease their pain. Talk about the power of suggestion: Patients in the second group needed less continued analgesia than those in the first group. We also know that chemotherapy is more effective when patients are told to visualize cancer cells being killed.

We need to use every available tool to support seriously ill patients, *especially* if the prognosis is poor.

The best way to help our patients is not to volunteer bad news, but to listen so well to their concerns that they truly feel they've been heard. We need to bring a humbleness to the bedside that allows the patient to tell us he's dying. We are never to tell him — unless he asks. And even then, the response must be supportive. For example, "The cancer has gotten very difficult to control, but you need to know that we're your team and we're going to see this through together."

I remind patients that they're in charge of their own lives and, even if things seem out of control, they have the power to decide which treatments they get and for how long. None of us can determine for another when it's time to let go.

— JOY UFEMA, RN, MS

- opportunity to communicate and discuss his impending death in a timely, honest, open manner with family, friends, and caregivers — people who will listen objectively and in a nonjudgmental manner
- excellent physical care, comfort, privacy, intimacy, sleep, and rest
- attentive management of pain and other symptoms that may change often
- permission to express his feelings openly, both positive and negative; permission to weep openly; and permission to express anger, resentment, and dissatisfaction as needed
- opportunity to explore the spiritual dimension of his life and to ask questions about mortality
- opportunity to discuss his preferences for funeral arrangements and the impact his dying process will have on his survivors.

Keep in mind that everyone has their own set of hopes. Yours will differ from your patient's. Typically, nurses in end-of-life care tend to hope for effective relief from unpleasant symptoms, a therapeutic relationship between staff and patient, a positive future for the patient and his family, a feeling of being valued, and the ability to redefine the goals of care as the illness progresses. By paying attention to your hopes and those of your patient and his family, you can help him achieve the satisfaction of reaching his end-of-life goals.

Providing information

Part of the ethical and clinical challenge of refocusing a patient's hope is determining how much information to provide and how often. Frankly, it's difficult and time-consuming to have repeated conversations about the patient's clinical status and the patient's and family's desire for information. The fact is, however, that doing so is as vital to successful end-of-life care as the relief of pain and other physical symptoms.

You need to find out and stay current with how much and what kind of information the patient wants so he can adjust his goals to fit the time he has left. His goal based on the information he had yesterday might have been to see his child graduate from college; his new goal based on information he receives today may be to live until his child's next birthday. He has every right to the information he needs to set such hopes.

The most helpful first step in communicating appropriately with patients, family members, and significant others during end-of-life care is to elicit their concerns. If needed, start by reviewing their understanding of the patient's clinical situation. Their explanations can help you gauge the amount and type of information they already have and what they'd like to receive during end-of-life care.

Pain relief is an especially important topic to investigate in detail. It's also important to understand how the patient and family members balance quality of life with length of life. It isn't terribly uncommon for family members to report feeling uninformed — even abandoned — by the patient's physician and, consequently, uncertain about how to handle these emotionally charged topics. You can help them find better ways to talk with the physician. By providing patients and families with the type and amount of information they want, you can help them reach a peaceful end of life.

Maintaining confidentiality

An important ethical consideration that emerges as information moves between patient, family members, and the palliative care team is the issue of confidentiality. You have ethical, legal, and professional obligations to maintain strict confidentiality of patient information. The American Nurses Association's Code of Ethics requires that you advocate for the patient's right to confidentiality and the related right to privacy.

As the protector of these rights, you must recognize that the need for end-of-life care doesn't justify unwanted intrusion into the patient's life. It also doesn't reduce the need for confidentiality. These are mandated by federal law.

The Health Insurance Portability and Accountability Act (HIPAA) was the first national legislation to ensure the protection of every patient's health insurance information. This law established standards and requirements for electronic transmission of health information. HIPAA protects the patient's right to the confidentiality of his medical information and imposes federal civil and criminal penalties for improperly using or disclosing protected health information.

Keep in mind that privacy and confidentiality are related but not synonymous. It's important to understand the difference between them so you can properly and ethically implement both concepts. (See *Understanding privacy and confidentiality.*)

The patient's rights, well-being, and safety should be paramount in making any professional decisions regarding the disposition of confidential information, whether it's oral, written, or electronic. Disclosure of this private information usually results from a trusting relationship in which the patient assumes that his information won't be revealed except in appropriate ways, such as for treatment, for payment of services, or for monitoring the quality of care being delivered.

Take care to be circumspect as you communicate with family members, significant others, friends, and concerned others, however well meaning their calls and inquiries. If needed, verify the identities of legal guardians or

Understanding privacy and confidentiality

In simple terms, privacy is about people, and confidentiality is about information.

Privacy is about a person's right to control the intrusion of others. In other words, it concerns what information you can have. As a nurse, you're accustomed to asking deeply personal questions in your effort to provide the best care possible. A patient's right to privacy means that he has the right to disclose details of his life, illness, feelings, finances, and family interactions — or not to disclose them. The patient always has the right to disclose no more than the demographic and insurance information required to obtain the service requested.

Confidentiality is about what you do with information you already know. Maintaining the patient's confidentiality is a well-recognized ethical standard in health care.

executors before providing information. If the patient chooses not to provide intimate details of his illness to certain family members, you must respect that choice.

To maintain the patient's privacy and the confidentiality of his health information, keep these points in mind:

■ Keep confidential all patient information, including name, diagnoses (physical and mental), current emotional state, financial status, and all demographic information, particularly his Social Security number.

■ Share patient information on a "need-to-know" basis according to medical necessity.

■ Avoid discussing patient information in public areas.

■ Avoid providing more information than is medically necessary, even to colleagues.

■ Keep confidential papers, computer disks, and other data in a secured area.

■ Don't allow confidential papers to remain in publicly accessible locations, such as on fax machines or copiers.

■ Technology, such as fax machines and e-mail, should be used only to support the patient's care and treatment. Verify the identity of anyone requesting information about a patient before you release it, and provide only essential information. Secure fax and regular mail are preferable to email or telephone contact.

■ Documents containing patient information should be shredded before being discarded.

Relieving pain

Another part of implementing end-of-life care is making decisions about pain relief. Patients and family members may wrongly believe that pain is inevitable and will become uncontrollable. Consequently, the patient may silently tolerate increasing pain, particularly in an attempt to deny his declining physical condition. Also, physicians may inadvertently erect barriers to the effective use of opioid analgesics. They may subtly convey that a "good" patient never complains or needs opioids. This places the patient in the position of attempting to please the physician and therefore withholding complaints of pain.

It's your ethical obligation to keep the patient's pain under control at all times during end-of-life care. The therapeutic goal is to lower the pain to a level that's acceptable to the patient. Uncontrolled pain will result in impaired sleep, reduced appetite, depression, anxiety, and possibly even thoughts of suicide as the pain becomes unrelenting. Unmanaged pain interferes with the dying person's ability to deal with unfinished business and address the spiritual aspects of dying.

Make certain that the patient and family members participating in his care have been thoroughly instructed in both drug and nondrug approaches to pain management. (See *Talking about pain management.*) Nondrug approaches include application of heat and cold, positioning, massage, relaxation techniques, distraction, imagery, and use of transcutaneous electrical nerve stimulation.

Many people — including some health care professionals — worry that a dying patient could become addicted to analgesics. Explain the difference between addiction, which is a psychological craving for a drug, and physical dependence, which means that uncomfortable symptoms develop if the drug is stopped suddenly. Also explain that it's normal for patients in pain to need increasing analgesic doses to keep the pain under control. This doesn't mean that they're addicted. On the contrary, it usually reflects an inadequate analgesic dosage.

Also, do your best to help dispel the myths and misconceptions held by many patients and family members. For instance, reassure them that many patients die without experiencing pain and that pain that does occur can be controlled quickly. Some patients fear that pain medications must be given by injection. Explain that some long-acting opioids are now available by mouth, in a transdermal patch, or by suppository.

The key to successful control of both acute and chronic pain in the patient who is receiving end-of-life care is repeated, comprehensive pain assessments. Unlike a person with acute pain, who may have such signs and symptoms as tachycardia, sweating, increased blood pressure, and facial gri-

Talking about pain management

Stress these points when talking with your patient about pain management.

■ Make sure you have all the information you feel you need to make informed choices about pain management.

■ Discuss various pain management options with your physician. Keep discussing until you're comfortable choosing among all the options.

■ Feel free to reevaluate your choices as your medical condition changes.

■ If you have pain, tell your physician and caregivers before it becomes severe.

■ Discuss your thoughts, concerns, and choices with family and significant others often.

■ If pain makes it difficult for you to do your usual household tasks, ask for help.

macing, a person with chronic pain may have such signs and symptoms as sleeplessness, withdrawal from family members and significant others, depression, or irritability.

 LIFESPAN Pain management in the elderly can be complicated by difficulties in pain assessment. Elderly patients may underreport pain, and physicians may attribute pain-related changes in physical activity to age. Elderly patients can be particularly susceptible to the adverse effects of nonsteroidal anti-inflammatory drugs, which can include gastrointestinal bleeding, diminished renal function, heart failure, and edema. Monitor patients carefully for sedation or confusion. And don't discount pain reports from cognitively impaired patients; these patients may not recall previous pain but usually can reliably report current pain.

Withdrawing treatment

Artificial nutrition and hydration can supplement or even replace ordinary nutrients by introducing a chemically balanced mix of nutrition and fluids through a tube placed directly into the stomach, upper intestine, or vein. Patients who don't receive these artificial nutrients and fluids undergo a natural process of reduced intake before they die. An important part of end-of-life care for patients who do receive this treatment will be the decision to withdraw the provision of nourishment and hydration.

Artificial nutrition and hydration can be a life-saving measure for a body attempting to heal itself. However, in end-of-life care, long-term use of tube feeding will neither reverse the course of the disease nor improve the quality of life. For some, even nutrition and hydration are considered extraordinary means of prolonging life, and it becomes the decision of the patient along with input from the family and the physician to stop these measures. To make certain that this is the wish of the patient himself, his wishes regarding artificial nutrition and hydration should be clearly stated in his advance directives.

The decision to withdraw nutrition and fluid, a painful one at best, becomes necessary when it's apparent to caregivers and family that prolonging life would only extend discomfort. (See *Discussing withdrawal of treatment*.) For patients in the final phase of illness, withholding food and fluids will not produce discomfort but instead will reduce the discomfort that results when fluid accumulates in tissues unable to excrete waste products.

 LIFESPAN A different set of ethical and legal issues emerge when the parent is to make medical decisions on their children's behalf.

This means that parents have the right to refuse life-sustaining medical treatment as long as such refusal doesn't constitute neglect. As the child's advocate, you'll need to make sure parents have received the information they need to make informed decisions. Remember that valid permission for diagnosis and treatment requires discussion of all treatment alternatives, including no treatment at all.

Rather than producing hunger and thirst in this type of situation, a side effect of starvation and dehydration will develop in which the change in metabolism and the resulting elevation of ketone level yields a mild form of euphoria. Deciding to give the patient nothing by mouth also eliminates the risk of aspiration.

 ALERT A high risk of aspiration can be determined by a swallowing study in a hospital; in a home setting, the risk of aspiration may be indicated by a tendency to cough, choke, or pocket food.

It's important to recognize that withdrawal or the withholding of treatment such as artificial nutrition and hydration isn't the equivalent of euthanasia. On the contrary, while euthanasia actively seeks to end the patient's life, withdrawal of treatment simply seeks to prevent further suffering that would be caused by prolonging the patient's disease process.

It's particularly important to clarify misconceptions. The family may assume that the patient's lack of appetite and poor hydration is causing the current disease process. Recognize the powerful emotional needs of family members to provide their loved one with food and water. Help them understand the uncomfortable effects of doing so once the patient is near death, and teach them to provide more appropriate comfort measures for the pa-

Discussing withdrawal of treatment

As the patient's death nears and it's time to talk about withdrawing nutrition and water, follow these steps.

■ Make sure you know the applicable policies of your institution and the laws of your state.

■ Choose a private setting where you won't be interrupted or distracted.

■ Find out what the patient and family already know about the patient's disease, prognosis, and treatment options; avoid using medical jargon.

■ Ask the patient and family to tell you which topics need more clarification.

■ Ask the patient to talk about his values and his goals of care; if he can't speak, ask the person designated by the patient to make medical decisions for him. If family members or significant others disagree about the goals of care, allow more time for explanation and discussion before discussing specific treatment decisions.

■ Find out if the patient and family have a timeframe in mind. Determine whether the physician has told them when the impending death is likely to occur. Talk about what can be done for the patient during the remaining time, focusing especially on comfort measures.

■ Progress through the conversation in small increments, and watch the family's reactions.

■ Let the patient and family express their emotions freely as they struggle with the reality of the situation. Have colleagues such as the facility chaplain, social worker, or hospice nurse available to assist if needed.

■ Reiterate the treatment strategy that the patient and family select.

tient, such as applying water-based gel to his lips, providing basic oral hygiene, reading scripture, holding his hand, or stroking his hair.

Many patients opt to spend their final days at home, with family, privacy, comfort, and control. Family members and significant others are more likely to stay intensely involved when a patient is receiving home care. Finally, home care tends to focus less on the illness and the "sick role" of the patient and more on the comforting details of daily living. No matter where your patient spends his final days, however, your attention to the ethical considerations of this difficult time will help the patient and his family make the transition with trust and care.

4 Legal considerations

If you're involved in end-of-life care, you'll be better able to act as an advocate for your patient and his family if you have a working knowledge of the legal considerations involved in this process. They stem largely from the Patient Self-Determination Act that was passed as part of the Omnibus Budget Reconciliation Act of 1990 and took effect in December of 1991. This Act requires health care providers to inform patients of their right to make their own health care decisions. The Act was intended to increase a patient's control over his own medical treatment decisions.

Informed decision-making

All health care agencies that receive Medicare or Medicaid funds are now required to provide written information to adults regarding their right to make medical decisions. Patients also must be given information regarding their right to formulate advance directives such as a living will and durable power of attorney for health care. The patient must be made aware of his right to decide about these issues when admitted to a hospital or skilled nursing facility, enrolled into a health maintenance organization, first receiving care from a hospice, or before receiving services from a home health agency. Legally, however, a health care agency cannot require a patient to sign an advance directive.

It's the responsibility of nurses to facilitate informed decision-making for patients making choices about end-of-life care. Your role in education, research, patient care, and advocacy plays a central part in the implementation of the Patient Self-Determination Act as end-of-life care begins. Make sure you understand the laws of the state in which you practice. It's your responsibility to make sure that your patient's advance directives are current and accurately reflect his choices. Promoting the self-determination of pa-

Advantages of advance directives

■ Peace of mind for the patient that his wishes will be carried out even if he can't communicate
■ Clear directions for family and significant others about the patient's wishes
■ Clear directions for health care providers about the patient's wishes
■ Prevention of family arguments and increased stress at an emotionally difficult time

tients regarding end-of-life decisions as well as acting as a patient advocate includes evaluating changes in the patient's perspective and current state of health. The nurse's responsibilities include facilitating informed decision making, a process that includes but isn't limited to advance directives.

Advance directives

Advance directives are a significant part of the requirements of the Patient Self-Determination Act. They include the living will, the durable power of attorney for health care, and the directive for organ donation. These are legal documents completed by competent adults that specify their choices regarding medical treatments if they become incapacitated. These documents also allow the patient to name someone to make choices for him if he can't make decisions on his own. These documents provide both legal and emotional advantages. (See *Advantages of advance directives*.)

The American Nurses Association recommends that several questions regarding advance directives be included as part of the admission process into any type of health care setting:

■ Do you have basic information about advance directives, including living wills and durable power of attorney?

■ Would you like to complete an advance directive?

■ If you already have an advance directive, may I have a copy of the document?

■ Have you discussed your end-of-life choices with your family and health care team?

Patients need to be informed that they can prepare their own advance directives, although state-specific documents should be used and witnessed. (See *Preparing an advance directive*, page 36.) Each state has its own witnessing requirement, with most requiring two adult witnesses. Some require a notary. Witnesses function to verify the patient's identity, make sure he wasn't coerced into signing, and confirm that he appeared to under-

Preparing an advance directive

Before your patient prepares an advance directive, suggest that he carry out these preliminary steps:
- Obtain information about the types of life-sustaining treatments available.
- If you are currently physically ill, obtain information regarding the expected progress of your disease.
- Discuss with your physician the expectations of your treatments and the risks of undergoing those treatments.
- Make sure your family and significant others are familiar with your value system and spiritual beliefs.
- Decide which treatments you would or would not want to receive.
- Document the types of treatments you would and would not like to receive if you can no longer communicate your wishes.
- Prepare several copies of the document and give one to your physician, your attorney, and your chosen surrogates. Keep a copy on hand for emergencies or future health care providers.

stand the process. Witnesses don't need to know the contents of the document they witness.

Requirements for who can witness an advance directive vary from state to state. In some states, the witness can't be related by blood or marriage, can't benefit from the patient's estate, and can't be a physician or employee of a health care facility in which the patient is being treated.

An advance directive remains in effect until it is revoked by the patient and can only be invalidated by completing a new advance directive. Therefore, an advance directive should be reviewed periodically to determine that it still reflects the patient's wishes.

Once the patient understands the importance of implementing advance directives, discuss the various types of these documents in detail.

Living will

A living will describes the treatments a patient does and doesn't want if he becomes incapacitated and has no chance of recovery. It usually authorizes the physician to either withhold or stop life-sustaining measures such as artificial ventilation, hydration, and nutrition. Your role in implementing a living will is to inform the patient of his options.

This is a crucial role. In 1997, only 15% of Americans had completed a living will. If a patient fails to complete a living will and then becomes unable to express his wishes regarding health care decisions, the medical staff may use their own discretion in deciding what type of medical care is most needed and most appropriate. They may ask for consent from a close relative, such as a spouse or adult child. However, these may not be the people most familiar with the patient's wishes, and personal and legal battles may ensue if family members and significant others disagree about the patient's wishes.

Assure the patient that a living will doesn't go into effect unless the patient can't make decisions for himself. Also, explain that it can be changed as needed, although states vary in their specifications regarding whether written or verbal notification is needed to change a living will. Assess and document the patient's mental competence to make health care decisions.

Legal immunity is provided to caregivers who comply with an appropriately prepared living will. There are situations, however, when a health care provider is permitted to reject a health care directive made either by a patient or the agent acting on his behalf. This can occur if:
■ the decision is objectionable to the conscience of the health care provider (See *Inappropriate intubation*, pages 38 and 39.)
■ the decision violates a facility policy based on reasons of conscience, as in the case of a hospital operated by a religious organization
■ the decision would perpetuate medically ineffective health care, or the care given would violate the generally acceptable health care standards then in use by the health care provider or the facility.

 LIFESPAN A patient's health care directives may be ignored completely in the case of pregnancy. If a patient is of childbearing age while completing a living will, she should explicitly state what she wants if that health care directive must go into effect while she is pregnant. Whether physicians will honor her directive will depend on the age of her fetus, the risks to mother and fetus, and the policies of the health care facility. During the second and third trimesters, the patient is likely to be given all medical care possible in an attempt to save both mother and fetus.

Usually, a living will is implemented either in terminal illness or permanent disability. The health care directive becomes effective when:
■ the patient is close to death from a terminal condition or is judged to be permanently comatose
■ the patient can't communicate his own wishes for his medical care—orally, in writing, or through gestures
■ the health care staff in attendance are notified of the patient's written instructions regarding his medical care.

The living will can prevent treatment from being implemented that will only extend life without restoring a comparable quality of life. The type, severity, and permanence or irreversibility of the disability need to be de-

EXPERT INSIGHTS

Inappropriate intubation

I work as the ombudsman in an ED. Last week the victim of a motor-vehicle crash was brought in and died within an hour. His granddaughter, who works in medical records, told me she was upset that the ED staff didn't intubate him to keep him "alive" until the family could get there. I told her that intubating a patient who can't survive isn't appropriate, but she didn't agree. What do you think? —W.D., Wis.

Without knowing all the circumstances, I agree with you. The staff shouldn't be asked to intubate a dying patient when treatment would be futile.

I experienced a similar situation involving a man in his early 50s who'd suffered a huge cerebral hemorrhage. Blood filled all four ventricles, and his right pupil was fixed and dilated. When he arrived at the hospital, he was unconscious, breathing on his own, but desaturating rapidly. His wife asked that he be supported on a ventilator long enough for his children to gather. She told me they'd arrive in about 6 hours.

I said gently, "I'm not sure Mark is going to live that long."

"But if you put him on the ventilator, he'll still be breathing when the kids get here," she protested.

"Sharon, even if we did intubate him, Mark's heart probably will stop soon after. Putting him on a ventilator isn't going to keep him alive."

fined as specifically as possible. If specific treatments are to be withheld when the patient can no longer speak for himself, the treatments should be described specifically.

Terms such as "extraordinary measures" or "life-sustaining care" are ambiguous and can be interpreted in various ways. Treatments that the patient views as prolonging life under intolerable conditions should be described specifically. For example, the patient may choose not to have a feeding tube inserted if he's in a persistent vegetative state.

Review the following medical treatments with the patient, and urge him to obtain additional information if needed and to discuss them with his health care provider and his family.

■ *Resuscitation.* Does the patient want cardiopulmonary resuscitation? Would he want it performed even if he were in the final stage of a terminal illness?

"I just want Mark's children to see him breathing," she said.

I took her hand and said, "I'm terribly sorry, but Mark is very close to death now. It would be inappropriate and unethical for the nurses and physicians and respiratory therapists to perform this procedure."

She began to choke back tears and pleaded, "I know he's going to die. I just want his sons and daughter to be here when it happens."

When she looked in my eyes, I must confess that I wavered for a moment. After all, Mark was in deep coma. Wouldn't it be a good thing for his children to say goodbye?

But I knew better. The severe brain injury that would stop his breathing would also stop his heart. It would be not only futile to intubate but also disrespectful to the patient.

I put my arm around her and shook my head "no." My heart ached for her, but I knew doing what she'd asked wouldn't be right, morally or professionally. "We don't have much time," I said. "Perhaps you want to spend it with your sweetheart. Let's go back to his room."

At her husband's bedside, she asked to be alone. A few minutes later, Mark died. When I went to her side, she looked up and smiled faintly.

"I told him he could go. I told him the kids and I would be okay."

And they are.

—JOY UFEMA, RN, MS

■ *Mechanical ventilation.* Does the patient want to be placed on a ventilator? If so, for how long? Would it matter to him what his prognosis was or if his condition was deteriorating?

■ *Nutrition and hydration.* Does the patient want to be fed artificially? If so, for how long? Would it matter to him what his prognosis was or if his condition was worsening?

■ *Dialysis.* Does the patient want to be dialyzed in the event of kidney failure? Would it matter to him if the treatment evolved into a permanent one rather than being temporary?

■ *Other end-of-life treatments.* These include antibiotics and analgesics. Does the patient want to receive these as palliative care if death is imminent?

Durable power of attorney

A durable power of attorney for health care, also known as a health care proxy, is a legal document that designates a person to make medical decisions for the patient if he can't communicate his wishes. If the patient has no relatives or significant others who can represent him and carry out his wishes appropriately, a health care provider other than the attending physician can be named as the surrogate decision maker. An attorney can also function in this capacity.

The need for a durable power of attorney for health care can be clearly seen in certain landmark court cases that influenced the concept. (See *The cases behind "the right to die."*) These cases graphically illustrate the emotional costs of long-term legal battles when a living will or a durable power of attorney for health care hasn't been completed.

Meeting the requirements

There are specific requirements for a durable power of attorney for health care to be properly functional:

■   The patient must be at least 18 years old or have been declared a legal adult.

■   The directive must be in writing, although it can be either typed or handwritten.

■   The document must be signed by the patient or, if he is unable to sign, can be signed by someone other than one of the witnesses of the document; in such a situation, the additional signer can do so only at the express direction of the patient and in his presence.

■   The document must designate an agent to make health care decisions for the patient when he is unable to do so and may designate another competent adult as a successor agent when the original agent is unable to implement his duties.

■   The document must specifically authorize the agent to make health care decisions for the patient if he is incapacitated. If the patient wants the agent to have the authority to withhold life-sustaining procedures or artificially administered nutrition and hydration, the document must specifically authorize these actions.

■   The document must have a date of execution and be witnessed and signed by at least two competent adults known by the patient or a notary public who is not the same person as the agent.

■   People who cannot serve as a witness to the proceeding include the patient's spouse, parent, child, grandchild, sibling, heir, attending physician, an employee of a life or health insurance provider for the patient, as well as the health care agent himself. No more than one witness can be the admin-

The cases behind "the right to die"

Nancy Cruzan

The phrase "right to die" was rarely heard before the 1983 tragedy of Nancy Cruzan. Injured in an automobile accident, she lay in a Missouri hospital in a vegetative state that was likely to continue for many years, sustained by artificial nutrition and hydration. The patient's parents, saying that their daughter would never wish to stay in such a state, petitioned the court to allow the hospital to withdraw the artificial fluid and nutrients. Although the Supreme Court denied the parents' request, eventually the case was retried in the Missouri courts and the Cruzans won. The Supreme Court ultimately concluded that citizens have a constitutional right to refuse treatment and that the right extends to a surrogate's interpretation of the patient's wishes if the patient can no longer express them. Nancy Cruzan died in 1990 after withdrawal of the feeding tubes.

Karen Ann Quinlan

In another well-known case, Karen Ann Quinlan suffered irreparable brain damage in 1975. In 1976, the New Jersey State Supreme Court ruled that she had the right to refuse life-sustaining medical treatment and that her rights could be implemented through surrogate decision makers, namely her parents. After her family waged a legal battle to remove her life-support equipment, she was removed from her respirator but continued to breathe unassisted. She remained comatose until she died in 1985 in a New Jersey skilled nursing facility.

Theresa Schiavo

A recent case involved Theresa Schiavo, who suffered severe brain damage in 1990 after her heart stopped. In 1998, her husband petitioned to have her feeding tube removed. Despite her parents' much publicized attempts to fight the request, the feeding tube was removed in March 2005. Theresa Schiavo died after 2 weeks without food and water.

istrator or employee of a health care provider who is caring for or treating the patient. Anyone who is already serving as surrogate decision maker for 10 or more patients is not allowed to serve as the health care agent.

The durable power of attorney must be made a part of the patient's medical record with the attending physician. It becomes effective when the patient is found to be incapable of making health care decisions. It continues in effect until it is revoked, until the patient dies, or until the patient is once again capable of making health care decisions.

A determination that a patient is no longer capable of making health care decisions must be made in writing by the attending physician. The cause and the nature of the incapacity must be documented. Notice of this determination must be given by the attending physician to the patient if the patient is able to comprehend the notice, to the person acting as the surrogate decision maker, and to the health care provider.

Once the surrogate has received notification, he or she must notify the next of kin unless the patient has specifically directed otherwise.

 LIFESPAN The surrogate decision maker has no authority to make any decision if the patient is known to be pregnant and the decision would likely result in the death of a fetus that would likely develop to the point of achieving live birth with application of appropriate health care.

Cultural considerations

In addition to the other issues that must be considered in an advance directive, cultural and religious factors may also need to be considered. Here's just one example: Conservative and orthodox Jews are encouraged to complete health care proxies that are aligned with Jewish religious law.

With the cooperation of its Commission on Legislation and Civic Action as well as many religious teachers, physicians, and attorneys, Agudath Israel of America, a nationwide branch of a worldwide organization of conservative Jews, has developed a health care proxy form that reflects Jewish law. Part of the form acts as a directive that the surrogate decision maker refer all questions to the rabbinic authority who the patient himself would consult were he able to do so.

Along with designating a person to make health care decisions when the patient cannot, there's a section for designating a specific rabbi to be consulted by the health care agent whenever questions involving Jewish law arise. If such a rabbi is unavailable or is unwilling to rule on a particular point, an orthodox Jewish organization or institution can be contacted to provide the proper rabbinic authority. According to Jewish tradition, preservation of life is considered to be paramount, surpassing all other commandments of the books of the Law.

Organ donation

Organ donation is more important than ever. According to the United Organ Sharing Network, the number of patients awaiting kidney transplants has almost tripled and the number of people awaiting liver transplants has increased tenfold since 1990. The process of organ donation and

Criteria for brain death

The Harvard Medical School Criteria for diagnosis of brain death as developed in 1968 are:
- Unresponsiveness
- Body temperature greater than 32° C
- Absence of depressant drugs
- No spontaneous movements
- Apnea (must be off the respirator for at least 3 minutes on room air)
- No reflexes, including fixed and dilated pupils and no decerebrate or decorticate posturing, swallowing, vocalization, corneal or pharyngeal reflexes, or stretch or deep-tendon reflexes
- Isoelectric electroencephalogram
- All of the above repeated after 24 hours

transplantation has advanced rapidly since the first successful transplant was performed by Dr. Joseph Murray in 1954. Advances in both immunosuppressant drugs and surgical techniques have increased the number of successful transplants as well as the quality of life for organ recipients.

Legal developments in the United States since World War II permit the procurement of organs after death from patients who choose to terminate life-sustaining medical treatments. These legal developments include the following:

■ *The Uniform Anatomical Gift Act of 1968.* This law allows patients older than age 18 to designate that their organs be transplanted after they are declared legally dead, although next of kin were given authority to both allow and refuse donation.

■ *Development of new criteria for death.* Also in 1968, a committee at Harvard Medical School chaired by Dr. Henry Beecher developed criteria for the determination of brain death. (See *Criteria for brain death.*) Basically, they required an irreversible failure of complete brain function, including brain stem function, in a person determined to be permanently comatose.

■ *The Uniform Determination of Death Act of 1981.* This legislation recognized irreversible lack of cardiopulmonary function and irreversible lack of entire brain function as legal definitions of death.

■ *Acceptance of precedent in allowing withdrawal of life-sustaining treatment.* All states now have either laws or precedents that recognize the Harvard Medical School criteria. Therefore, once a donor meets either cardiopulmonary or neurologic criteria for death, he can be legally used as an organ donor.

Obtaining consent

Many people—including physicians, nurses, and especially family members—are understandably anxious about allowing organs to be procured from a patient after withdrawal of life support, even if the patient clearly asked that his organs be donated. Family members have the authority to accept or deny organ donation, unless the patient signed an organ donor card, had "organ donor" added to his driver's license or state ID card, or registered with his state's online donation registry. Even with legal documentation or consent, hospitals typically request surrogate consent from family members. Next-of-kin priority order when no legal evidence of consent is present or the hospital wishes to confirm consent is:

- spouse
- adult son or daughter
- either parent
- adult brother or sister
- guardian at time of death
- any other authorized person.

The most important criterion for consent is the family's knowledge of the patient's wishes regarding organ donation before he becomes unconscious. This decision may be complicated by family members who are unfamiliar with the patient's wishes or have hesitations based on their own values. Consequently, organ procurement organizations have developed policy changes that mandate respecting the consent of a patient if the specific state's legal process has been completed. This permits the procurement of donated organs without requiring additional consent from family members.

Best practice states that the organ procurement organization (OPO) staff should approach the family of a potential donor, together with a member of the health care team, only after the OPO determines that the patient is a viable donor. Only OPO providers trained in the progression of the organ donation process should approach families regarding the possibility of donation. Organ donation should never be discussed with the family until these steps have been followed.

Pronouncing death

Historically, the medical profession has been given the responsibility for identifying the moment when death occurs. When a medical practitioner is unable to certify death, then the responsibility falls to the coroner. This would occur, for example, when there is no body available for assessment. Legally, death must be certified for several reasons, including:

- statistical and epidemiological purposes
- for distributing property to survivors

- for burial to take place
- for criminal law purposes when death occurs during the commission of a crime.

Ethically and legally, organ procurement can't begin until a donor has been declared dead. However, as medical practitioners, we know that this process isn't always clear and simple. For example, how can we be certain that either neurologic or cardiopulmonary criteria for death have been satisfied and that subsequent function has been irretrievably lost? Is cardiac arrest irreversible if circulation could be restored but no resuscitation efforts will be made? Or is cardiac arrest irreversible only when circulatory function can't be restored despite resuscitation efforts? These issues, once raised, are not easily dismissed.

One of the first protocols for organ procurement after controlled death was developed at the University of Pittsburgh and is known as the Pittsburgh Protocol. This protocol requires a two-minute wait after cardiopulmonary arrest before organ procurement can begin on the assumption that a two-minute period precludes spontaneous resumption of circulatory or respiratory function after arrest. However, the scientific validity of this argument has been questioned because the phenomenon of autoresuscitation has never been studied in depth.

Understanding conflicts

Because organs are removed after circulatory arrest, donors are referred to as Donors after Cardiac Death (DCD) donors. This type of organ donation can occur only after family members of a patient with irreversible brain death agree to the needed withdrawal of ventilatory support. Family members then are approached regarding the option of donation. After consent is obtained, the patient either will stay in the intensive care unit or will be transferred directly to the operating room for ventilatory support to be withdrawn. The attending physician will witness cardiopulmonary arrest. Then, 2 to 5 minutes, depending on hospital protocol, must pass before the procurement procedure can begin.

DCD organ donation may engender legal and ethical conflicts. For example, there can be a conflict between ensuring organ viability and waiting for cardiovascular cessation after neurologic cessation is verified and life support withdrawn before procurement begins. A goal of organ transplantation is to minimize the warm ischemia time (time when the organs are still warm, needing high levels of oxygen, and getting none) of transplantable organs. This can be reduced by cannulation of the femoral artery and infusion of a cooling liquid into the abdominal cavity before the patient is removed from artificial life support. However, this procedure can't be performed without the consent of family members and may feel to the family like an invasion of a body that, because of the effects of artificial life support, seems to still be alive. Furthermore, the termination of life support and the potential conflict of interest between the provision of care and organ recovery provide other avenues of inquiry. To help avoid this conflict of interest, the members of the patient care team are completely separate from the members of the organ procurement team.

Finally, conflicts may arise over the use of controlled versus uncontrolled donation in DCD donors. In a controlled DCD donor procedure, the team withdraws ventilatory support, waits for cardiopulmonary arrest, and then rapidly procures organs before they can physically deteriorate. In an uncontrolled DCD, or commonly called deceased donor procedure, the patient dies suddenly, can't be resuscitated, and — with family consent — tubes are inserted to instill cold fluid to preserve the organs until they're procured. Although a few states allow instillation of cooling fluid while awaiting family consent, the procedure is rarely performed because of the ethical questions involved in failing to obtain consent and respecting the patient's body after death.

Despite these potential conflicts and the emotional repercussions of end-of-life care, the decision to donate organs can benefit the patient and his family by generating a sense of community, feelings of life continuing on as a cycle, and the knowledge that others will benefit from this gift and the patient's life.

PART TWO

Caring
for patients

5 | Evidence-based care

The philosophy that underlies palliative care is relatively simple: to minimize suffering and maximize quality of life. At the end of a patient's life, palliative care replaces curative care.

However, although it may be easy to understand the general philosophy of palliative care, it's much harder to know how to deliver high-quality palliative care during a patient's final months, weeks, days, and hours. This is in part why certain organizations have begun creating guidelines for care.

One such organization is the National Consensus Project for Quality Palliative Care, which actually is a consortium of several palliative care associations. Another is the World Health Organization, which has proposed palliative care guidelines with international application.

National Consensus Project for Quality Palliative Care

The National Consensus Project for Quality Palliative Care currently includes three major palliative care organizations:
- American Academy of Hospice and Palliative Medicine
- Hospice and Palliative Nurses Association
- National Hospice and Palliative Care Organization.

In 2004, in response to the growing need for end-of-life care, this group plus the Center to Advance Palliative Care and the Last Acts Partnership created *Clinical Practice Guidelines for Quality Palliative Care* for palliative care providers, including nurses, in a range of treatment settings. More than 100 experts in palliative care contributed to these evidence-based guidelines. The purposes of the guidelines are to:

- facilitate development and continuous improvement of clinical palliative care programs
- establish definitions of essential elements in palliative care that promote quality, consistency, and reliability
- establish national goals for access to quality palliative care
- foster performance measurement and quality improvement in palliative care
- foster continuity of palliative care across settings, including hospitals, residential care facilities, hospice, and the patient's home.

The guidelines promote quality, consistency, and reliability of services. They also promote access to palliative care across care settings. To help clinicians incorporate the guidelines into practice, the organization identified eight areas of particular concern. (See *Eight aspects of palliative care*, page 50.)

Structure and processes of care

This topic stresses the importance of using an interdisciplinary assessment of patient and family to form the plan of care. The assessment should include:

- a physical examination
- review of the patient's medical records
- review of laboratory data, tests, and procedures
- discussion with providers about the patient's diagnosis, prognosis, and appropriateness of end-of-life care or a referral to hospice.

During the assessment, make sure to investigate the patient's and family's expectations, their goals for the patient's life and care, their understanding of the patient's disease and prognosis, and their preferences for the type of care the patient will receive and where that care will take place.

 LIFESPAN Always consider the developmental needs of the patient and family, including pediatric patients and the children and grandchildren of adult patients.

When developing a care plan, solicit input from:

- the patient
- his family, caregivers, and chosen friends
- his health care providers, including the palliative care team and related specialists
- his chosen spiritual advisers.

Always keep in mind that patient and family preference should underlie the types of care and the services the patient receives. Make sure you respect the patient's cultural and religious values and integrate them into the plan of care. The palliative care team should communicate at least weekly to review the plan, staffing needs, quality of care, and clinical practices that affect the patient and family. Also, the palliative care team should coordinate respite and volunteer services for families and caregivers.

Eight aspects of palliative care

Caring for dying patients requires clinical expertise in widely varying aspects of life and health. The National Consensus Project for Quality Palliative Care has identified these eight topics as the framework for the organization's clinical practice guidelines:

- Structure and processes of care
- Physical aspects of care
- Psychological and psychiatric aspects of care
- Social aspects of care
- Spiritual, religious, and existential aspects of care
- Cultural aspects of care
- Care of the imminently dying patient
- Ethical and legal aspects of care

National Consensus Project for Quality Palliative Care (2004). *Clinical practice guidelines for quality palliative care.* http://www.nationalconsensusproject.org.

 ALERT If the patient receives end-of-life care at home, make sure the patient and family can reach appropriate staff around the clock, 24 hours a day, 7 days a week.

If the patient receives care away from home, the palliative care team must ensure the patient's safety, flexible visiting hours, appropriate space for family meetings, and privacy. Referrals to specialists and community services may be needed based on the needs and preferences of both patient and family. Likewise, the staff will need access to emotional support, educational resources, and continuing professional education—and should document their use.

This aspect of the guidelines also includes evaluation of palliative care programs by patients, families, health professionals, and community members to help maintain continuous quality improvement and identify and promote helpful changes. This process helps the important goal of integrating evidence-based research and quality procedures and policies into palliative practice.

Physical aspects of care

The guidelines specify that physical aspects of care must be delivered by professionals trained and skilled in managing the symptoms of terminal illness, which commonly include:

- anorexia
- anxiety

- confusion
- constipation
- depression
- fatigue and weakness
- insomnia
- nausea
- pain
- shortness of breath.

You'll need to provide ongoing assessment, including assessment of any adverse effects of treatment and changes in the patient's functional ability.

The guidelines stress that symptom management should be based on the best available clinical evidence and should focus on the safe and prompt reduction of symptoms for as long as they last. Keep in mind that the patient is the one who determines his level of tolerance for symptoms. Treatment should be tailored accordingly. It may include drug, nondrug, and complementary or supportive therapies. Make sure to address the patient's physical, psychological, social, and spiritual dimensions in the treatment plan.

Teach the patient and family about the patient's disease and its prognosis, expected symptoms, the patient's level of functional impairment, treatments that may help, and the adverse effects of treatments. Also, teach family members how to keep the patient safe and how to provide comfort measures. In particular, teach about the importance of pain management. Many people—including some health care providers—are anxious about opioid analgesics. They fear that opioids will cause addiction, heavy sedation, and an earlier death. However, when a patient is receiving end-of-life care, these fears inappropriately take the focus off the patient's comfort and quality of life. (See *Putting the patient first*, pages 52 and 53.) Make sure you have a risk management plan that addresses the use of controlled substances for long-term symptom management and that it's reviewed and implemented by the palliative care team.

Psychological aspects of care

A patient with a terminal illness may develop depression, anxiety, delirium, cognitive impairment, and other psychological problems. Family members will face psychological challenges as well. As part of palliative care, perform a psychological assessment of the patient and his family. Make sure they understand the patient's disease and its prognosis, the signs and symptoms he probably will have, expected treatments and their adverse effects, the patient's need for care, and helpful coping strategies. Take care to identify patients and family members at risk for grief and bereavement. If the patient is elderly, pay special attention to assessing for depression and comorbid complications.

EXPERT INSIGHTS

Putting the patient first

Sometimes when I care for terminally ill patients, I feel overwhelmed by competing demands — the patient's wishes, the family's priorities, the physician's decisions. Is there any easy way to sort through the conflicts? — M.E., Calif.

The clearest path is simply to focus on being the patient's advocate, never giving up until we've exhausted all efforts to ease her suffering and keep her comfortable. The following story illustrates my point.

The first time I met Lydia, who had end-stage chronic obstructive pulmonary disease, she was sitting upright in a chair surrounded by her husband and two grown daughters. Struggling to breathe, she was diaphoretic and pale. Her profound shortness of breath was unrelieved by supplemental oxygen.

I knelt down by the chair and said, "Lydia, I know you'd rather use your energy breathing than talking, so I'll just ask you one or two questions." Are things getting rough now?"

She nodded yes.

"And what do you want from us?"

"Relieve...my...suffering," she gasped, her eyes pleading.

I told her that I could make her much more comfortable and that I'd check her chart and call her physician. She reached for my hand and kissed it.

A quick scan of the Kardex revealed that Lydia previously had been receiving 4 mg/hour of morphine I.V., but that the physician had reduced the dosage because of sedation.

While I was reading the Kardex, Lydia's nurse asked if we should just give lorazepam (Ativan) to decrease anxiety.

Use your assessment of the patient's and family's stress, anticipatory grieving, and coping strategies to guide interventions. Teach and help the family to provide safe, appropriate psychological support to the patient, and make sure they have means of support as well.

Interventions for psychological distress may include drug, nondrug, and complementary therapies. Your goal is to address the patient's and family's psychological needs and to support their emotional growth, healing, reframing, completion of unfinished business, and bereavement. It's common for the bereavement component of palliative care to extend a full year, sometimes longer, after the patient dies.

"No," I replied. "She's anxious because she can't breathe. What she needs to be comfortable is a higher dose of morphine — at least 4 mg/hour and probably a bit more."

After talking with the physician, I documented his new order — including morphine titrated "to comfort" — and explained the plan of care to my patient.

"When I increase the morphine, Lydia, you're going to get sleepy and sedated. Is that okay with you?"

"Are you saying she's never going to wake up?" blurted her daughter.

"I...don't...want," Lydia gasped.

"She doesn't want to be sedated like that. Isn't that right, Mom?"

Shaking her head, Lydia looked up at me and said emphatically, "I...don't...want...to...wake...up."

Both daughters and her husband began to cry, but Lydia did not.

I told them we'd increase the morphine just enough for Lydia to get relief. If that dosage sedated her, then that would be the maximum amount she'd receive. But if she lost relief, we'd increase the dosage again until she was comfortable.

Once again Lydia took my hand and said, "I...need...more...now."

I slowly titrated the morphine. At 8 mg, Lydia lay back in the chair and relaxed. This was the first time in days she hadn't needed to sit upright to breathe. She feel asleep for several hours and awoke with a smile for her family.

Later, when Lydia was discharged home with hospice, I was grateful for all the teachers who'd taught me lessons about palliative care — foremost among them, patients like Lydia.

— JOY UFEMA, RN, MS

Social aspects of care

Palliative care also should focus on the many social needs of patients and their families during end-of-life care. (See *Assessing social needs*, page 54.) For example, the care plan should identify possible caregiver strain and ways to reduce it. The patient and family — members of the interdisciplinary team — should be invited to attend weekly meetings about the patient's care. The team also may coordinate meetings at the patient's home to answer patient and family questions, help with decision-making, discuss the goals of care, and offer support.

Assessing social needs

The social needs of a patient and family can be wide-ranging and warrant a detailed assessment. Focus on supporting the family as a unit and also on individual members in their many family roles. Some of the areas of social assessment identified by the National Consensus Project for Quality Palliative Care include:

- access to needed equipment
- access to nutritional products
- access to prescription and over-the-counter drugs
- access to transportation
- caregiver availability
- community resources, including school and work settings
- family structure and geographic location
- finances
- legal issues
- lines of communication
- living arrangements
- medical decision making
- perceived social supports
- relationships
- sexuality and intimacy
- social and cultural networks
- work and school settings.

National Consensus Project for Quality Palliative Care (2004). Clinical practice guidelines for quality palliative care. http://www.nationalconsensusproject.org.

Spiritual, religious, and existential aspects of care

The guidelines also urge the palliative care team to assess and address the spiritual issues that patients and their families are likely to experience. Some of the spiritual or life concerns that commonly arise in end-of-life care are:

- life review
- hopes and fears
- the meaning or purpose of life
- beliefs about afterlife
- guilt and forgiveness
- tasks needed to feel that life is complete.

Make sure the patient has access to his preferred clergy or spiritual advisor. Also, take steps to make the patient comfortable expressing his religious preference and displaying any religious or spiritual symbols that have meaning for him—even if they differ from your own. Likewise, the palliative care team should facilitate any religious or spiritual rituals desired by the patient or family, especially when the patient dies.

Cultural aspects of care

The next section of the guidelines stresses the need to accommodate the patient's and family's language, dietary preferences, and ritual practices. When interacting with the patient and family, take care to communicate your respect for their cultural preferences. If possible, make sure the care team includes staff who speak the patient's and family's preferred language. If that's not possible, use an interpreter if needed.

Care of the imminently dying patient

As the patient develops signs and symptoms of impending death, the guidelines urge you to communicate that development appropriately to the patient, family, and staff. The care team will need time to prepare for and manage the increased intensity of care the patient will need during this phase. Also, make sure to document all changes in the patient's symptoms. And encourage the patient and family to explain their wishes about where the patient will die.

Ethical and legal aspects of care

Finally, the guidelines specify that, if the patient is able to make decisions, those decisions should guide the care plan and the family's level of involvement in his care. If he can no longer make decisions and communicate them, you'll need to rely on advance directives; the patient's previously expressed wishes, values, and preferences; and appropriate surrogate decision makers. When possible, urge patients and families to finalize their advance directives, wills, guardianship agreements, and other legal documents before the patient becomes unable to express his wishes.

If ethical concerns arise, handle them according to the principles of beneficence, self-determination, confidentiality, and informed consent. Keep patient and family care consistent with the nurse's professional codes of ethics. The entire palliative care team should be involved in such ethical issues as withholding nutrition and hydration, adopting "do not resuscitate" orders, and giving sedatives.

Naturally, members of the palliative care team must be knowledgeable about medical decision making, regulatory issues, advance care planning, and appropriate use of controlled substances. Also, make sure you understand and can take part in pronouncing death and inquiring about organ donation and autopsy.

By attending to each of the eight areas identified in the *Clinical Practice Guidelines for Quality Palliative Care*, you can help promote quality and consistency in palliative care while giving patients and families the best possible quality of life at the end of life.

World Health Organization

The World Health Organization (WHO) is the United Nations agency for health. Its goal is for all the world's people to have the highest possible level of health. In 2003 through 2005, the WHO published *Integrated Management of Adolescent and Adult Illness*. The four-part guidelines reflect the expert opinions and practices of an international working group and include modules that address acute care, chronic HIV care, general principles of good chronic care, and palliative care.

The palliative care guidelines are divided into the following areas of instruction:
- assessment and treatment
- management of pain
- preventive interventions for all patients
- management of key symptoms
- special considerations
- end-of-life care.

Assessment and treatment

This section starts by reviewing three areas of assessment important for patients receiving palliative care. First is a "quick check" that includes assessing the patient's airway, breathing, and circulation and checking for chest pain, severe abdominal pain, neck or severe head pain, and fever from a life-threatening cause. It then suggests assessing the patient for coughing or trouble breathing, for undernutrition or anemia, for mouth or throat problems (such as thrush or ulcers), and for pain.

Also, make sure to provide appropriate assessment and treatment if the patient complains of fever, diarrhea, genitourinary or lower abdominal symptoms, anogenital lesions, a skin problem or lump, a headache or other neurologic problem, a mental problem, nausea or vomiting, contractures or stiffness, constipation or incontinence, or hiccups.

General treatment steps include teaching the patient and family how to give appropriate palliative care at home, keeping the patient as much in charge of his own care as possible, providing prescribed drugs and other techniques to manage pain and other symptoms, making sure the patient and family have the supplies they need, giving them written instructions as needed (including prescribed drugs and their indications and dosages), making sure they know when to call for help, and making appropriate referrals for them.

Managing pain

Pain management is particularly important in end-of-life care. Start by determining the cause of the patient's pain. Ask if the pain is new or changed. Assess the type of pain, such as bone pain, nerve pain, or muscle spasm. Find out whether the pain has a mental or spiritual element. Finally, use a standardized assessment tool to help determine the pain's severity.

To guide treatment, the WHO uses an analgesic ladder. (See *The analgesic ladder*, page 58.) As possible, give analgesics by mouth (or rectum), give them on a schedule rather than as needed, and link the first and last doses with waking and sleeping times. Start with a small dose and adjust it against the pain until the patient is comfortable. Give the next dose before the current one wears off. And be prepared to give rescue doses if the patient has breakthrough pain between scheduled doses.

Special types of pain may need unusual treatments. For instance, nerve pain may respond to amitriptyline. Or, for muscle spasms, the patient may receive diazepam. Pain also may respond at least in part to nondrug treatments. They include:

■ psychological, spiritual, and emotional support and counseling to address issues of guilt, fear of dying, loneliness, anxiety, and depression

■ answering the patient's questions and explaining what's happening to help relieve fear and anxiety

■ touch, such as stroking, massaging, rocking, or vibration

■ deep-breathing and relaxation techniques

■ distraction, including through music or imagery

■ prayer

■ traditional or cultural practices that aren't harmful to the patient.

Another important aspect of managing pain is managing the adverse effects of analgesics, which may include constipation, respiratory depression, itching, and urine retention. Make sure to teach the patient and family about pain medication, potential adverse effects, and alternate methods for pain control.

Preventive interventions

Preventive interventions should be taught to all patients. They include oral care, measures to prevent pressure sores, safety precautions for bathing, and methods to prevent contractures. Also, the WHO guidelines suggest teaching patients and family members how to perform range-of-motion exercises

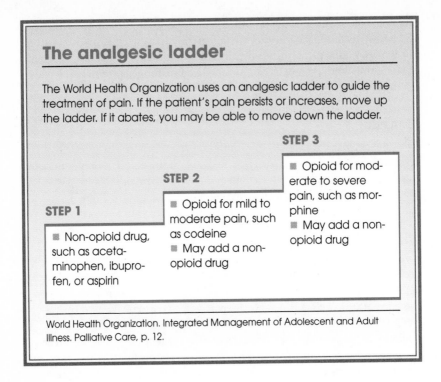

The analgesic ladder

The World Health Organization uses an analgesic ladder to guide the treatment of pain. If the patient's pain persists or increases, move up the ladder. If it abates, you may be able to move down the ladder.

STEP 1
- Non-opioid drug, such as aceta-minophen, ibupro-fen, or aspirin

STEP 2
- Opioid for mild to moderate pain, such as codeine
- May add a non-opioid drug

STEP 3
- Opioid for moderate to severe pain, such as morphine
- May add a non-opioid drug

World Health Organization. Integrated Management of Adolescent and Adult Illness. Palliative Care, p. 12.

and how to correctly transfer a weak patient. These precautions help prevent injuries not only to the patient but also to caregivers.

Managing key symptoms

This section of the guidelines provides specific measures to manage the symptoms that arise most commonly during end-of-life care. Such symptoms include:

- anxiety and agitation
- confusion
- constipation
- cough
- depression
- diarrhea
- difficulty breathing
- dry mouth
- fever
- hiccups
- incontinence of urine or stool
- insomnia
- itching

- mouth ulcers or painful swallowing
- nausea and vomiting
- pressure sores
- rectal tenderness
- vaginal discharge
- weight loss.

The guidelines include common drug treatments and their usual dosages. They also offer home-care remedies that may be implemented easily by the patient and family. For example, if the patient has insomnia, the suggested home care includes reducing noise, giving pain medication if appropriate, reducing caffeine intake late in the evening, and listening to the patient's fears and anxieties that may be contributing to the insomnia.

Special considerations

This section focuses on patients with special needs, such as those with HIV or AIDS and children with terminal illnesses. It reviews precautions against infection, sexuality issues, and adverse effects of antiretroviral drugs. It also offers effective communication tips to help assess and manage pain in children and addresses the importance of support for and from caregivers, family, siblings, and school friends of pediatric patients.

End-of-life care

Finally, the guidelines emphasize the importance of psychosocial and spiritual support for dying patients and their families. They advise providing active listening, counseling, empowerment, and help as the patient and family prepare for the patient's death. Teach the family how to keep the patient comfortable near the end of life by such actions as moistening the patient's lips, mouth, and eyes to prevent dryness. Explain the signs of imminent death to help ease the family's anxiety as the patient declines. And make sure the patient and family have access to bereavement counseling.

Both sets of palliative care guidelines discussed in this chapter offer proven techniques for helping to maximize the comfort and quality of life of dying patients and their families. In chapters to come, you'll find specific advice to help you care for patients with such terminal illnesses as cancer, heart failure, amyotrophic lateral sclerosis, chronic obstructive pulmonary disease, and end-stage renal disease.

6 Palliative drug therapy

Almost invariably, dying patients receive many drugs and undergo various degrees of organ failure before reaching the end of life. Both of these issues will complicate your ability to manage the patient's symptoms and maximize his level of comfort through the dying process. This is particularly true when the patient is a child, for whom drug dosages aren't always established. (See *Drug precautions in children*.)

Naturally, the more drugs a patient is receiving, the more likely he is to experience adverse effects and drug interactions. Plus, physiologic changes common to dying patients—such as a slowed metabolism, impaired renal or hepatic function, poor circulation, and an impaired central nervous system (CNS)—may raise the risk of drug accumulation and toxicity. Also, de-

---

Drug precautions in children

Children absorb, metabolize, and excrete drugs differently than adults do. These differences may alter the amount of a drug needed to produce a therapeutic effect and the amount that causes toxic effects. Because standardized dosages commonly aren't available for children, follow these tips:
- Evaluate the child's kidney and liver function.
- Avoid using the child's age to make assumptions about organ system development.
- In lean children, use height to calculate doses.
- In larger or obese children, use body surface area or the next higher dose.

hydration and electrolyte imbalances can affect how drugs are absorbed by the body.

Despite these challenges, with carefully orchestrated drug therapy and close attention to the pharmacokinetics and pharmacodynamics of the drugs involved, you can ease many or all of the symptoms experienced by dying patients. And by preparing and teaching caregivers how to use an emergency drug kit, you can ensure that even a patient dying at home can receive time-ly customized palliative drug therapy. An emergency kit contains a selection of drugs commonly needed by dying patients and is available for immediate use as symptoms arise. (See *Contents of an emergency kit.*)

Symptoms experienced most often by patients in end-of-life care include pain, fatigue, dyspnea, excessive respiratory secretions, nausea and vomit-ing, constipation, and diarrhea. This chapter offers a quick overview of the best ways to manage these symptoms through careful drug therapy.

Contents of an emergency kit

Drug	Form	Uses
morphine *Alternative:* oxycodone (Roxicodone, Oxyir)	Oral, sublingual, or rectal	Pain Dyspnea
lorazepam (Ativan) *Alternative:* diazepam (Valium)	Oral, sublingual, or rectal	Seizures Anxiety Muscle spasm Agitation
hyoscyamine (Levsin) *Alternative:* scopolamine (Scopase, Transderm Scōp)	*hyoscyamine:* oral or sublingual transdermal patch or oral	Excess secretions Nausea and vomiting if patient has GI ob-struction
haloperidol (Haldol)	Oral or rectal	Agitation Nausea and vomiting
lorazepam (Ativan), diphen-hydramine (Benadryl), halo-peridol (Haldol), and meto-clopramide (Reglan), com-pounded as ABHR	Rectal or troche	Nausea and vomiting
prochlorperazine (Compazine)	Oral or rectal	Nausea and vomiting
phenytoin (Dilantin)	Oral	Seizures

Pain

Pain is the problem that most dying patients and their families worry about most. When it's inadequately managed, pain can affect a person's ability to sleep, cope, and relate to others. It dramatically affects quality of life, and it will affect the patient's quality of death.

Although many nondrug treatments—such as massage, relaxation exercises, and acupuncture—can help reduce a patient's pain, the mainstay of pain management is drug therapy. Depending on the severity and cause of the pain, some drugs may offer more benefits or fewer adverse effects than others. Drugs commonly used to manage pain in a dying patient include nonopioids, opioids, and some other drugs that are effective in certain situations. Keep in mind that some common drugs shouldn't be used at all during end-of-life care.

Nonopioids

Usually, pain control starts with a nonopioid, such as acetaminophen or a nonsteroidal anti-inflammatory drug (NSAID). (See *Common nonopioid analgesics*, pages 64 and 65.) Acetaminophen's mechanism of action isn't known exactly, but the drug probably works centrally. Aspirin and NSAIDs inhibit cyclooxygenase, which decreases prostaglandin production and, in turn, pain and inflammation. Acetaminophen and opioids decrease pain but not inflammation.

Acetaminophen has few side effects, but the dosage may be limited by hepatic impairment, which may increase the risk of hepatotoxicity and liver damage. NSAIDs may increase the risk of peptic ulcer, renal failure and edema, allergic reactions, and hearing loss. They also may increase the risk of hemorrhage.

 LIFESPAN Because of its safety profile, acetaminophen is the preferred drug for treating chronic pain in elderly patients. Don't give more than 3 grams daily, and avoid acetaminophen entirely if the patient consumes excessive amounts of alcohol. Make sure the patient's liver function is checked periodically.

Consider these age-related changes whenever you add or adjust a drug:
■ Renal and hepatic function may be decreased even if an elderly patient isn't in end-stage organ failure.
■ An age-related decrease in lean body mass may influence drug metabolism and availability. If the drug is lipid-soluble (such as fentanyl), it may have a slightly delayed onset and increased risk of accumulation; if it's water-soluble (such as hydromorphone and morphine), the opposite may occur.
■ Decreased gastric motility may delay absorption of NSAIDs and increase their adverse gastrointestinal (GI) effects.

Opioids

If the patient has severe pain, he'll need an opioid. Morphine is the archetypal drug in the class. It's highly effective and available in many forms, including sustained-release capsules, immediate-release tablets, concentrated liquids, suppositories, and subcutaneous and intravenous injections.

Morphine and similar drugs (such as oxycodone, hydrocodone, diamorphine, and fentanyl) all have a similar influence on cerebral opiate receptors. They also may produce similar adverse effects, such as these:

■ Up to 1 in 3 patients starting morphine may have nausea and vomiting. Usually, it abates after a short course of antiemetics.

■ Pruritus may develop; if it does, you may need to switch the patient to a different opioid.

■ Constipation develops in almost all patients who take opioids. Usually, a laxative — such as lactulose, senna, or docusate — is prescribed along with the opioid.

■ Morphine and other opioids may cause respiratory depression, hallucinations, and sedation, all of which may be distressing for both patient and family. As the patient adjusts to the dosage, this effect usually remits, although it may recur briefly whenever the dosage is increased. Make sure to differentiate this drug-related effect from progression of the patient's disease.

Opioid doses may be limited by toxicity, which you should suspect if the patient is confused and has myoclonic jerks and pinpoint pupils. However, as long as toxicity isn't evident, there's no ceiling for the opioid dosage in a dying patient. (See *Merciful meds*, page 66.) When used appropriately, opioid analgesics are safe and effective, with little risk of addiction.

 ALERT Many analgesics combine an opioid with a nonopioid to increase pain relief. A common combination is Acetaminophen and codeine. For a dying patient in severe pain, the limiting factor for many of these combination drugs is the nonopioid part. For the patient to receive enough benefit from the opioid, he'd need an overdose of the nonopioid component. These drugs are best used for mild to moderate pain.

Other drugs

Pain comes in many forms and from many sources. Likewise, drugs used to relieve pain work by many different mechanisms. (See *How drugs reduce pain*. page 67.) Matching the drug's mechanism of action with the type of pain you're trying to relieve can increase your success. In fact, some types of pain respond best to drugs that aren't even known as typical analgesics. For example:

■ In a patient with brain cancer, pain may stem from pressure inside the skull. This pain may respond best, initially at least, to high doses of dexamethasone (Decadron), a corticosteroid.

Common nonopioid analgesics

Class	Generic name	Available forms and strengths
P-Aminophenol derivatives	acetaminophen	*Tablets:* 80 mg, 325 mg, 500 mg, 650 mg *Suppositories:* 120 mg, 125 mg, 325 mg, 600 mg, 650 mg *Liquid:* 160 mg/5 ml, 500 mg/15 ml *Elixir:* 80 mg/2.5 ml, 120 mg/5 ml, 160 mg/5 ml, 325 mg/5 ml
Salicylates	aspirin	*Tablets:* 325 mg, 500 mg, 650 mg, 800 mg *Suppositories:* 120 mg, 200 mg, 300 mg, 600 mg
	choline magnesium trisalicylate	*Tablets:* 500 mg, 750 mg, 1,000 mg *Liquid:* 500 mg/5 ml
Proprionic acids	ibuprofen	*Tablets:* 100 mg, 200 mg, 300 mg, 400 mg, 600 mg, 800 mg *Suspension:* 40 mg/ml, 100 mg/5 ml
	naproxen	*Tablets:* 250 mg, 375 mg, 500 mg *Suspension:* 125 mg/ml
Acetic acids	indomethacin	*Capsules:* 25 mg, 50 mg *Extended-release:* 75 mg *Suspension:* 25 mg/5 ml *Suppositories:* 50 mg
	diclofenac	*Tablets:* 25 mg, 50 mg, 75 mg, 100 mg *Extended-release:* 100 mg
	nabumetone	*Tablets:* 500 mg, 750 mg
Pyranocarboxylic acids	etodolac	*Capsules:* 200 mg, 300 mg *Tablets:* 400 mg, 500 mg *Extended-release:* 400 mg, 600 mg
Cyclooxygenase-2 inhibitors	celecoxib	*Capsules:* 100 mg, 200 mg, 400 mg

■ A patient with severe mouth ulcers may respond to a preparation that contains viscous lidocaine, a short-acting anesthetic.
■ A patient with chronic neuropathic pain may respond to carbamazepine (Tegretol) or gabapentin (Neurontin), both of which are anticonvulsants. Both are modestly successful at relieving neuropathic pain.

Starting dosage	Maximum daily amount
2,600 mg/day given q 4 to 6 hours	6,000 mg
2,600 mg/day given q 4 to 6 hours	6,000 mg
1,500 mg for one dose; then 1,000 mg q 12 hours	4,000 mg
1,600 mg/day given q 4 to 6 hours	3,200 mg
500 mg/day given q 8 to 12 hours	1,500 mg
200 mg/day given q 8 to 12 hours	200 mg
150 mg/day given q 8 to 12 hours	225 mg
1,000 mg/day given q 24 hours	2,000 mg
600 mg/day given q 6 to 8 hours	1,200 mg
200 mg/day given q 12 to 24 hours	800 mg

■ Painful neuropathies may also be treated with clonidine (Klonopin), other alpha$_2$ agonists, mexiletine (Mexitil), and other local anesthetic analogues.

■ Tricyclic antidepressants, especially amitriptyline, seem to reduce neuropathic pain by acting centrally.

EXPERT INSIGHTS

Merciful meds

Which drugs do you give most often to keep patients comfortable at the end of life? — M.L., Arizona

Controlling pain is a priority for a dying patient. Oral morphine (which also helps control dyspnea) is the analgesic of choice because it doesn't become toxic and you can easily adjust the liquid form as needed. For example, if the patient wants to be more alert for certain events (such as a family visit), you can adjust the dose down. You may need to adjust the dose up before repositioning him.

Give lorazepam (Ativan) with morphine if the patient becomes agitated. It's our responsibility to manage the patient's anxiety and confusion, as well as pain, at the end of life.

Inspired air flowing across accumulated respiratory secretions can cause what's commonly called the death rattle. Hyoscyamine sulfate (Levsin Drops), an anticholinergic drug, decreases secretions and minimizes this sound, which can be especially distressing to family members. Place the drops inside a comatose patient's cheek.

Don't forget to maintain good mouth care throughout your patient's life, even if he's unconscious. Frequent mouth cleaning with a Toothette dipped in mouthwash can remove debris and odor, allowing a more pleasant experience for those who wish to offer him a final kiss.

— JOY UFEMA, RN, MS

■ Another psychotropic drug may help as well: tetrahydrocannabinol and some other cannabinoids, either as marijuana from the *Cannabis sativa* plant or as a synthetic drug. Many patients report substantial pain relief, particularly from marijuana, but the use of cannabis derivatives is illegal in many countries.

Inappropriate drugs

Some drugs that you might expect to use during end-of-life care aren't, in fact, appropriate for dying patients. One of the most common is propoxyphene, which is included in Darvocet and some other combination analgesics. It's widely used for moderate pain, especially in long-term care set-

How drugs reduce pain

Drug class	Mechanism of action
Alpha agonists	Inhibit release of substance P, a polypeptide that works as a neurotransmitter
Anticonvulsants	Block influx of sodium ions, preventing depolarization and generation of an action potential
Corticosteriods	Block production of prostaglandins
Gamma-aminobutyric acid (GABA) agonists	Increase release of GABA, an inhibitory neurotransmitter in the brain
Local anesthetics	Block influx of sodium ions, preventing depolarization and generation of an action potential
N-methyl-D-aspartate receptor antagonists	Inhibit binding of excitatory amino acids, such as glutamate, preventing transmission
Nonsteroidal anti-inflammatory drugs	Block production of prostaglandins
Opioids	Bind with opiate receptors and block release of substance P
Tricyclic antidepressants	Prevent reuptake of serotonin and norepinephrine

tings. However, it isn't appropriate during end-of-life care — especially for elderly patients — because it causes sedation, confusion, and dystonia.

Meperidine (Demerol) is another poor candidate for ongoing pain control, for several reasons. It causes buildup of a toxic CNS metabolite known as normeperidine, it has a short duration of action, and it has extremely poor oral bioavailability. These characteristics yield a high risk of adverse effects and a relatively weak analgesic effect compared to other opioids. Consequently, this drug is best used to relieve short-term, acute pain, such as pain caused by a surgical procedure.

Also inappropriate for use during end-of-life care are opioid agonist-antagonists, which promote analgesia at some opiate receptors while simultaneously reversing that effect at other receptors. Examples include nalbulphine (Nubain) and butorphanol (Stadol).

Fatigue

Fatigue, like pain and anxiety, is a subjective word used to describe wide-ranging sensations. Examples include:

- being easily tired or exhausted
- having decreased energy or trouble maintaining a usual level of activity
- feeling generally weak
- struggling to concentrate or remember
- reacting in a more emotional way than usual.

At one time, fatigue was considered almost inevitable in patients receiving end-of-life care, particularly cancer patients. It's also common in patients with human immunodeficiency virus (HIV) infection, cardiac disease, and many other terminal illnesses. Now we know that fatigue may stem from many different sources, including the drug regimen that's designed to help the patient feel better.

No matter how close your patient is to death or which treatments he's receiving, it's important to assess the causes and possible treatments of his fatigue. For example, it could result from anemia, decreased intake, emotional distress, infection, or the effects of his drug regimen or disease process. No matter what its cause, severe fatigue profoundly interferes with quality of life and the patient's ability to function adequately in his final days.

Because fatigue is a multidimensional symptom, it's crucial that you adequately assess and identify its origins and effects. Consider whether fatigue is a primary symptom, what may be causing it, and whether its therapeutic management is reasonable given the risks and benefits to the patient.

A number of interventions are available to help ease the patient's fatigue. For example, corticosteroids may decrease fatigue in cancer patients. Although the mechanism of action is unknown for this purpose, it may be their euphoriant effect that helps corticosteroids to decrease fatigue. Avoid long-term use of corticosteroids because they lead to metabolic abnormalities, osteoporosis, myopathies, and increased risk of infection.

Megestrol acetate can improve fatigue and general well-being within about 10 days in terminally ill patients. The suggested dose is 160 to 480 mg every day. The mechanism of action is unclear, but it may be related to glucocorticoid or anabolic activity and effects on cytokine release. This drug also improves appetite in some patients.

Thalidomide and omega-3 fatty acids can help manage cachexia and may decrease fatigue as well. In patients with advanced HIV disease, thalidomide helps preserve the ability to function in daily activities.

Anemia

Always assess for anemia if a patient complains of fatigue. Severe anemia, with a hemoglobin level less than 7 g/dl, usually warrants a blood transfusion. In patients undergoing chemotherapy, epoetin alfa may help reduce fatigue. A typical dosage is 10,000 units three times weekly increasing to 20,000 units three times weekly depending on the patient's response. The main disadvantages of epoetin alfa are the cost and the 4- to 8-week delay before the hemoglobin level increases by 1 to 2 g/dl and symptoms improve.

Depression

If your patient's fatigue is related to depression, he may need an antidepressant. A selective serotonin reuptake inhibitor (SSRI) probably is a better choice than a tricyclic antidepressant because SSRIs tend to have fewer adverse effects.

Sedation

If fatigue stems from opioid-induced sedation, the patient may benefit from a psychostimulant, such as methylphenidate (Ritalin), pemoline (Cylert), or dextroamphetamine (Dexadrine).

Dyspnea

Dyspnea becomes more likely—and more distressing—as the end of life approaches. Between 50% and 70% of dying patients experience it, sometimes with profound shortness of breath, copious secretions, fatigue, and coughing. The patient and family may find this development deeply frightening.

Often, dyspnea in a dying patient has no clear cause. Many end-of-life complications can cause it, such as infections that cause fluid to accumulate around the lungs. Fluid also may accumulate around the heart (pericardial effusion) or in the abdomen (ascites). Several medical treatments may contribute to dyspnea; for example, fluids given to maintain hydration and nutrition may interfere with breathing by causing unintentional fluid accumulation in the lungs and abdomen. (See *Causes and treatments of dyspnea,* pages 70 and 71.)

If the underlying cause of your patient's dyspnea is intravenous fluids, you may need to stop them. Adding oxygen therapy may help, especially if you humidify the oxygen to help the patient breathe more restfully. Also, try elevating the patient's head a bit, and either cool the room air or use a

Causes and treatments of dyspnea

Cause	Assessment findings	Treatment
Chronic obstructive pulmonary disease	■ Wheezing, rhonchi on auscultation ■ Persistent cough ■ Chronic shortness of breath	■ Nebulized bronchodilators ■ Corticosteroids ■ Morphine
Excess secretions	■ Congested sensation ■ Audible secretions in upper airway and bronchi on auscultation ■ Productive cough	■ Positioning: side-lying with elevated head of bed or semi-prone ■ Anticholinergic, such as scopolamine (Scōp TD), hyoscyamine (Levsin), or atropine
Heart failure	■ Progressive dyspnea ■ Rales on auscultation ■ Jugular vein distension	■ Diuretics ■ Morphine ■ Inotropic drugs ■ Activity and diet consideration as appropriate for quality of life
Pleural effusion	■ Distant or absent breath sounds in lower fields, most often unilateral ■ Progressive shortness of breath	■ Positioning: head of bed elevated ■ Morphine ■ Thoracentesis, with or without sclerosing therapy if appropriate for quality of life
Pneumonia	■ Fever ■ Productive cough ■ Rhonchi or consolidation on auscultation	■ Acetaminophen or ibuprofen for fever ■ Positioning and anticholinergics to control secretions ■ Antibiotic therapy if desired for quality of life
Pneumonitis (treatment-related)	■ Increasing chronic shortness of breath ■ Cough	■ Morphine ■ Nebulized bronchodilators ■ Corticosteroids

(continued)

Causes and treatments of dyspnea *(continued)*

Cause	Assessment findings	Treatment
Superior vena cava syndrome	■ Acute shortness of breath ■ Jugular vein distension ■ Swelling of neck and face	■ Emergency radiation therapy ■ High-dose corticosteroids ■ Morphine
Tumor or other obstruction	■ Breathlessness ■ Areas of decreased aeration on auscultation, possibly with localized rhonchi if fluid or secretions are trapped by obstruction ■ Cough	■ Oral morphine ■ Nebulized bronchodilators or corticosteroids ■ Positioning ■ Radiation or chemotherapy if advancing tumor is suspected

fan to help create a gentle breeze. Each of these actions can help the patient feel better able to breathe.

Certain drugs can help ease the patient's work of breathing as well, including diuretics, opioids, anxiolytics, bronchodilators, and corticosteroids.

Diuretics

For patients with evidence of hypervolemia—such as dyspnea, crackles, and peripheral edema—a diuretic such as furosemide (Lasix) may help decrease fluid volume, vascular congestion, and cardiac workload. Furosemide can be given by mouth, intravenously, subcutaneously, or intramuscularly.

Opioids

An opioid such as morphine can help ease the struggle to breathe. If the patient isn't already taking morphine daily, start with 5 to 6 mg every 4 hours. If the patient already takes morphine for pain, increase the dose by 50%.

Anxiolytics

Anxiolytics, such as benzodiazepines and phenothiazines, can help relieve the psychological distress and autonomic responses that may accompany dyspnea. They can depress hypoxic and ventilator responses and may alter the patient's emotional responses to dyspnea. Keep in mind, however, that these drugs are poorly tolerated in long-term therapy, are metabolized by the liver, and produce long-acting metabolites.

The anxiolytics most often used to treat dyspnea are lorazepam (Ativan) and diazepam (Valium). Phenothiazines such as chlorpromazine (Thorazine) and promethazine (Phenergan) may be helpful for patients who have anxiety with dyspnea. Combining one of these drugs with morphine may be especially helpful because phenothiazines have anticholinergic effects that reduce respiratory secretions and provide antiemetic effects.

Bronchodilators

Bronchodilators decrease the work of breathing. Most are categorized as sympathomimetic nonselective or selective adrenergic drugs. (See *Treating dyspnea with bronchodilators.*) Patients with both pulmonary disease and cardiac disease may benefit from a nonselective agonist. However, excessive use of beta-adrenergic drugs may cause cardiac stimulation and be harmful in elderly patients who have cardiac disease.

Corticosteroids

Although their use isn't fully established, corticosteroid therapy may start when bronchodilators become ineffective. Corticosteroids may help reduce dyspnea by decreasing inflammation and increasing bronchodilation.

Respiratory secretions

As death nears, patients may develop excess secretions in the upper and lower airways, producing what's commonly known as a death rattle. Conditions of the lungs or neck, pneumonia, heart failure, and renal failure all increase the risk of this disconcerting symptom.

Secretions can be reduced by giving an anticholinergic, such as hyoscyamine (Anaspaz or Levsin Drops) or transdermal scopolamine (Transderm Scōp). Hyoscyamine is less costly than scopolamine and has less sedative effect. These anticholinergics have largely replaced atropine injections, which were once common. Make sure the patient receives frequent mouth care to offset the drying effects of anticholinergics.

Coughing can be persistent and uncomfortable and can lead to respiratory distress or increased secretions. It may be caused by the patient's drug regimen, smoking, lung disease, or an irritable diaphragm. If your patient is coughing, consider giving the expectorant guaifenesin, either alone in high-dose form (Humibid L.A.) or with codeine for suppression (Robitussin A-C). Phenergan in various combinations or benzonatate (Tessalon) provide other options.

Treating dyspnea with bronchodilators

Class	Uses	Route and dosage
Nonselective agonists		
epinephrine	Acute bronchoconstriction	*Subcutaneous:* 0.2 to 1 mg q 4 hours p.r.n.
Epinephrine inhaler, Primatene, Vaponefrin	wheezing, bronchocon- striction, asthma	*Inhaler:* 1 puff (200 mcg) q 3 to 4 hours p.r.n.
Nonselective beta agonists		
isoproterenol	*Isuprel:* intraoperative bronchospasm	*I.V. push:* 0.2 mg (1 ml) in 10 ml normal saline solution or 5% dextrose; then 0.01 to 0.02 mg (0.5 to 1 ml) p.r.n. *Sublingual:* 10- to 15-mg tablet p.r.n.
	Isuprel: chronic bron- choconstriction, asthma	*Inhaler:* 1 to 2 puffs (130 mcg each) up to five times daily p.r.n.
	Isuprel inhaler: bron- choconstriction in asthma, chronic obstructive pul- monary disease (COPD)	*Nebulizer:* 5 to 15 deep inhalations of 10-mg/ml solution
ethylnorepinephrine	Acute bronchospasm	*Subcutaneous, I.M.:* 1 to 2 mg (0.5 to 1 ml) p.r.n.
Selective beta$_2$ agonists		
albuterol sulfate	*Proventil, Ventolin:* bron- chodilation in asthma, COPD	*Inhaler:* 1 to 2 puffs (90 mcg each) q 4 to 6 hours *P.O.:* 2 to 4 mg q 3 to 4 hours; maximum, 8 mg q.i.d.

(continued)

Treating dyspnea with bronchodilators (continued)

Prototype	Uses	Route and dosage
Selective beta$_2$ agonists (continued)		
albuterol sulfate (continued)	Alupent: bronchodilation for COPD	Inhaler: 3 to 4 puffs q 3 to 4 hours p.r.n.; maximum, 12 puffs daily Nebulizer: 10 deep inhalations of undiluted 5% solution q 4 hours p.r.n. P.O.: 10- to 20-mg tablets t.i.d. or q.i.d.

Nausea and vomiting

Nausea and vomiting arise in about 40% of terminally ill patients, possibly contributing to loss of appetite, physical and mental problems, esophageal tears, and reopening of surgical wounds. Uncontrolled nausea and vomiting also may interfere with the patient's ability to take drugs and receive other treatments.

Chemotherapy and radiation therapy administered for stomach or brain cancer are common causes of nausea and vomiting in patients receiving end-of-life care. In chemotherapy, there are three types of nausea and vomiting: anticipatory, acute, and delayed. The anticipatory form may occur before or during chemotherapy. The acute form usually occurs within 24 hours after chemotherapy. The delayed form typically occurs more than 24 hours after chemotherapy and lasts several days. Delayed nausea and vomiting can cause serious illness. Patients receiving radiation therapy for stomach cancer may develop nausea and vomiting because the cells of the GI tract are very sensitive to radiation; radiation to the brain probably stimulates the vomiting center.

Nausea and vomiting sometimes can be controlled with nondrug therapies, such as changing the patient's diet or using hypnosis or guided imagery. Sometimes these therapies can change the patient's view of chemotherapy. However, antiemetic drugs of several different types are the mainstay of therapy. (See *Drugs for nausea and vomiting*.) They may be used alone or in combination. A 5-HT$_3$ receptor antagonist, such as ondansetron, is the most effective choice for many patients.

Drugs for nausea and vomiting

Drug class	Drug name
Antiemetics	▪ granisetron (Kytril) ▪ haloperidal (Haldol) ▪ ondansetron (Zofran) ▪ prochlorperazine (Compazine)
Antihistamines	▪ diphenhydramine (Benadryl) ▪ hydroxyzine (Atarax)
Anxiolytics	▪ lorazepam (Ativan)
Cannabinoids	▪ dronabinol (Marinol)
Cholinergics	▪ metoclopramide (Reglan)
Corticosteroids	▪ dexamethasone (Decadron) ▪ prednisone (Deltasone)

If the patient is scheduled to receive an emetogenic therapy, such as chemotherapy, make sure to give the antiemetic beforehand. You'll need to keep antiemetic levels constant in the patient's blood to control nausea and vomiting effectively. Also, keep in mind that anticipatory nausea and vomiting often don't respond to antinausea drugs because the vomiting center in the brain isn't directly triggered. In this situation, anxiolytic drugs may be more effective.

Some patients find cannabinoids helpful, especially for chemotherapy-induced nausea and vomiting. Two forms are available. A synthetic form of delta-9-tetrahydrocannabinol (THC), the active ingredient in marijuana, can be prescribed as an antiemetic for patients who haven't responded to other treatments. It's called dronabinol (Marinol). The other form is the marijuana plant, an illegal substance that some patients take by mouth or smoke.

Constipation

Constipation is a common problem for patients in end-of-life care, usually resulting from drug therapy, often from opioids. However, many factors may contribute to constipation in patients with terminal diseases. (See

Causes of constipation

In a terminally ill patient, opioid therapy isn't the only thing that can cause constipation. Here are some other common causes.
- Diet and hydration, especially if impaired swallowing decreases food and fluid intake
- Chemical imbalance, particularly hypercalcemia and hypokalemia
- Intestinal compression, which can develop in patients with cancer that affects the abdomen
- Psychosocial concerns, such as fear, anxiety, and depression, which increase epinephrine release and, in turn, decrease peristalsis
- Immobility caused by fatigue, pain, or disease effects, which decreases normal gastrointestinal motility

Causes of constipation.) If possible, the better course is to prevent constipation rather than treat it.

Most palliative care programs routinely employ a stepped bowel regimen. The regimen typically starts with a combination drug, such as Senokot-S (senna combined with a stool softener), for daily use. If the patient still doesn't have regular bowel movements, this drug may be increased or the bowel regimen can step up to a stronger drug, such as bisacodyl (Dulcolax), lactulose (Chronulac), magnesium hydroxide (Milk of Magnesia), or magnesium citrate. (See *Drugs for constipation.*)

If the patient's constipation results from opioid therapy, subcutaneous infusion of metoclopramide may be effective. Opioid-induced constipation also may respond to oral use of naloxone, an opioid antagonist. Because opioid effects on the GI tract are mediated by peripheral opioid receptors, first-pass hepatic metabolism of oral naloxone yields little systemic availability, which lets naloxone antagonize the GI peripheral opioid receptors without significantly antagonizing CNS opioid receptors. The result: a laxative effect without withdrawal symptoms or breakthrough pain.

Untreated or inadequately treated constipation can advance to bowel obstruction. Fleet or other enemas, glycerin or bisacodyl (Dulcolax) suppositories, and manual disimpaction may be needed to remove hardened stool.

Drugs for constipation

Type	Effects	Drugs
Stool softener	■ Mixes fat and water in small and large intestines to soften stools	■ docusate sodium (Colace)
Bulk-producing laxative	■ Holds water in stool to maintain bulk, which stimulates peristalsis in the small and large intestines	■ calcium polycar-bophil (Fiberall, FiberCon) ■ methylcellulose powder (Citrucel) ■ psyllium (Natural Fiber Metamucil)
Hyperosmotic laxative	■ Holds fluid in the colon, lowering pH and increasing peristalsis	■ glycerin ■ lactulose (Cephulac) ■ sorbitol
Saline laxative	■ Attracts and holds water in the colon, increasing pressure in the small and large intestines and stimulating movement	■ magnesium citrate ■ magnesium hydroxide (Milk of Magnesia) ■ sodium phosphate (Fleet Phospho-soda)
Stimulant laxative	■ Acts directly on intestinal mucosa of the colon or nerve plexus; alters water and electrolyte secretion	■ bisacodyl (Dulcolax) ■ senna (Senokot, Senolax)

Diarrhea

Diarrhea may result from drugs, foods, fecal impaction, or the patient's disease process. Diarrhea can predispose the patient to dehydration, electrolyte imbalance, and skin breakdown. Loperamide (Imodium, Kaopectate) given after each bowel movement typically can control diarrhea; however, more persistent episodes may warrant giving diphenoxylate and atropine (Lomotil). Patients with HIV-related diarrhea may need injected drugs, such as octreotide (Sandostatin).

No matter which combination of symptoms a dying patient develops, your skillful use of drug therapy is essential in helping maintain the patient's dignity and prevent suffering. Understanding the principles of drug therapy and how they can be customized for end-of-life care will help you manage your patients' end-of-life symptoms wisely and well.

7

Psychosocial, spiritual, and cultural care

In end-of-life care, no matter what the patient's particular diagnosis, the goal of the palliative care team is to relieve the patient's symptoms and help the patient and family resolve issues that may be blocking the way to a peaceful death. Providing this kind of care requires much more than simply attention to the patient's physical symptoms. It requires your ability and willingness to interact with the patient and family about deeply emotional issues. And it requires respect and sensitivity for spiritual and cultural aspects of the patient's life.

Psychosocial care

Psychosocial care at the end of life is a critical aspect of the palliative care process. Three of the most common psychosocial developments that need your care are grief, anxiety, and depression.

Grief

Grief is one of the most pervasive emotions produced by loss, dying, and death. (See *Definitions of loss*.) Since psychiatrist Elisabeth Kübler-Ross introduced her five-stage model of loss (denial, anger, bargaining, depression, and acceptance) in 1969, others have developed models that describe grief. These models share several traits:
- Grief is a process.
- Grief includes a variety of intense emotions.
- Grief can result in a new level of emotional organization.
- A new identity is often gained at the end of the grief process.

Definitions of loss

Loss is a real, perceived, or anticipated taking away of something. The loss can be physical, symbolic, or social.

Grief encompasses the mental, physical, social, and emotional responses to loss.

Mourning is the outward, social expression of a loss — part of the process of adapting to the loss.

Bereavement is the period of grief and mourning. It includes the inner feelings and outward reactions of the survivor.

Grieving process

The grieving process starts long before the patient's actual death and is known at that point as anticipatory grief. Grief takes many forms and requires ongoing assessment of both patient and family — starting the moment a patient learns he has a terminal condition.

Grief may be accompanied by many other emotions, including depression and anxiety, which also need assessment and follow-up. Factors that influence the grief response include age, culture, prior losses, the quality of the relationship with the dying person, the time to prepare for the death, and the resolution of past issues.

Grief responses are highly individualized and dependent in part on personal coping skills. In certain circumstances, grief may become chronic, delayed, exaggerated, or masked. This is known as a complicated grief reaction. (See *Risk factors for complicated grief reactions*, page 80.) Social workers sometimes have official responsibility for monitoring patient and family coping status. However, it's an ongoing task of the entire palliative care team to identify and manage risk factors for particular difficulties and complications as a patient grieves his situation and the family grieves their impending loss. Keep in mind that some family members experience great relief when the suffering of their loved one ends in death.

Honest communication

Maintaining open lines of honest communication with the patient and family members is a central part of palliative care and is critical to developing a trusting relationship. Giving the patient and family some control over the time, place, and content of each discussion helps to build trust and rapport.

Risk factors for complicated grief reactions

Low-level risk factors
■ Trouble communicating with the palliative care team
■ Family conflict
■ Extreme dependency
■ Legal or financial issues
■ Signs of spiritual distress, such as expressing feelings of being abandoned by God

High-level risk factors
■ Family members who express difficulty coping with previous deaths
■ Patient or family isolated from their support system by geography
■ Lack of close relationships
■ History of violence
■ Signs of inadequate coping skills
■ Signs of substance abuse or mental health issues

At times, the patient may want to talk only with you about the impact of his terminal illness. At other times, he may want you to lead the whole family in a discussion that helps them clarify their own responses to the loss.

If possible, set aside uninterrupted time to be with the patient. (See *Finding time to talk.*) Help the patient clarify his issues of loss and explore his feelings at a deeper level. Practice being comfortable with periods of silence, and don't rush to fill gaps in the conversation. (If this is difficult for you, try role playing with another nurse.) Sometimes, patients may need your silence and a caring presence more than a discussion.

Anxiety

Anxiety is another of the most common emotions experienced by both patients and family at the end of life. Often, the anxiety relates directly to uncertainty about the manner and time of death. As the dying person begins to experience significant changes in bodily function and loss of family roles, fear may increase.

 ALERT Certain drugs can cause anxiety as well, including corticosteroids, bronchodilators, and antihistamines.

Assessment
Usually, asking directly is the best way to determine the level of the patient's anxiety. You also may be able to observe some evidence. Common

COMFORT & CARE

Finding time to talk

To help a patient and family with their grief, you'll need time to talk—
a precious commodity not only for nurses but for patients battling the
physical effects of end-stage illness. Try these ideas to help maximize
the quality and quantity of your talk time.

■ Organize the patient's daily routine to include periods of uninterrupted time.

■ Plan discussions during times when the patient has the highest energy level.

■ Ask the patient if he needs time to talk. Find out if he'd like other
family members to be present. Then set a time when all of you can attend. Keep in mind, however, that not all conversations can be
planned in this way.

■ Ask the patient to keep a journal about his experience of being ill.
Then, when you talk together, he can refer to the journal if needed.

■ Start a quality assurance project that assesses institutional support
for spending quality time with patients.

indicators of anxiety include muscle tension, irritability, and obsessive
statements or behaviors. Some patients may deny being anxious but display
these signs. Others will openly express their fears and may even complain
of feeling panicked or out of control of their emotions around their loved
ones.

Management
You and the entire palliative care team can help the patient and family cope
with anxiety by exploring how they've successfully coped with stress in the
past. Encourage the patient to recall examples, especially humorous ones, of
past problems and how the patient handled them. These interventions can
serve both as opportunities for reminiscing about past life accomplishments
and reminders that anxiety can be overcome.

Other interventions that the team can use to help the patient manage
anxiety include reassuring the patient and family that anxiety is common
and manageable. Reinforce the use of behavioral strategies that the patient
has used in the past to cope with anxiety (prayer, family discussions, jour-
naling, humor, distracting and pleasurable activities such as family visits
and movies or books). Suggest complementary therapies, such as massage,
meditation, or music. Another great antidote for anxiety is exercise or physical activity if the patient is able.

When a patient's anxiety is beyond the level of self-management strategies, an anxiolytic — usually a benzodiazepine — may be helpful.

Depression

Depression is common among dying patients and their family members, and it may be difficult to distinguish from the normal grief that accompanies loss and bereavement. Often, the only difference between grief and depression is the intensity and length of the expression of sadness.

A patient with an end-stage illness may experience depression for many reasons, including the advanced effects of the illness, poorly controlled pain, adverse drug effects, substance abuse, unresolved psychosocial issues, and a family history of mental health problems. (See *Treating emotional symptoms.*) Screen for depression in every patient. If you suspect it, conduct a thorough assessment of the patient's physical and psychological condition.

Assessment

During initial and ongoing assessments, look for indications that a patient or family members could be experiencing depression. Common signs and symptoms include:

- hopelessness
- despair
- thoughts of suicide
- lack of participation in daily routine
- sleeplessness
- loss of appetite and weight.

Various approaches are available to screen for depression. If you aren't using a standardized tool, use simple but direct questions as your assessment. Even a question as simple as, "Do you feel depressed?" can be very effective in assessing a patient's level of depression.

Management

The management of depression in palliative care patients includes both drug and psychological therapy. Drugs may include selective serotonin reuptake inhibitors (SSRIs), tricyclic antidepressants (TCAs), and other psychostimulants. SSRIs are safer and have fewer adverse effects. However, it may take weeks for either SSRIs or TCAs to provide significant therapeutic effects. Psychostimulants such as methylphenidate (Ritalin) or dextroamphetamine (Dexedrine) may be more useful for providing better quality of life when time is short. Corticosteroids such as prednisone have a euphoric effect and stimulate appetite; they may be useful in short-term situations. Nondrug interventions include supportive counseling, spiritual counseling, and ongoing monitoring of the patient's mental state. Complementary ther-

EXPERT INSIGHTS

Treating emotional symptoms

*I'm caring for a home hospice patient who's terminally ill with gastric
cancer. His physical symptoms are under control, but he seems to
have a restlessness in his soul. When I ask if he has any unfinished
business, he turns away without answering. His wife says she thinks
he's thinking about a son from his first marriage. They had a falling
out years ago and haven't spoken since. I don't want to butt in, but intuition tells me this rift needs to be resolved for his own peace of mind.
What's your advice? –S.T., Ontario*

I admire your self-restraint. You might be tempted to telephone the
son, but that would violate your patient's privacy and overstep your
role, no matter how well-intentioned you might be.

I suggest asking the patient's wife to join you at the bedside.
Explain that you're aware of the break in his relationship with his son;
then ask if he'd like to talk about it. Also offer to leave if he wishes to
speak privately with his wife about it.

If he declines to discuss this with you, remind him that you care
about his comfort, both physical and emotional, and that if he ever
does feel like talking — about anything — you're available.

This isn't the time to gather up your sphygmomanometer and walk
out the door. Instead, continue your assessment in a warm, dignified
way while making small talk or discussing how much fluid he's been
drinking. You want to promote a sense of acceptance and trust, regardless of whether he chooses to confide in you.

If, however, he rolls to face you and his wife and begins to share his
feelings, sit down, touch his arm, and give him your undivided attention.

Recently, a lovely woman I knew only casually asked me to help
with her terminally ill dad. Dana explained that the physician had said
that her dad was depressed and had also recommended another
round of chemotherapy. But her dad had turned down treatment for
cancer or depression and seemed to be willing himself to die by refusing to eat or drink.

"Is anything else going on that could be making him feel so hopeless?" I asked.

Dana then revealed that her dad had left her family when she was
a child. He'd come back into her life after her mom died 3 years ago.
"It's kind of hard for me to let him go now that I care about him," she
admitted.

(continued)

Treating emotional symptoms *(continued)*

"So you love your dad, Dana?" I asked.

"Yes, I guess I do."

"Does he know that?"

"I haven't said it in so many words, but I think he knows."

I suggested that she go in and tell him all the things in her heart. "Then we'll ask him what he wants," I said.

An hour later, I was paged to her father's room. "Oh, Joy," she sobbed. "I told him I loved him and forgave him. He opened his eyes and said, 'I accept your forgiveness, and I love you too.' Then he just rolled back on the pillow and died!"

I have to admit that I was a bit stunned.

"Dana, you gave your dad two wonderful gifts today: Your loving forgiveness and permission to be relieved of his burden of guilt. This is powerful stuff."

She smiled and gave me a big hug.

I hope your work with your troubled patient is as rewarding for you.

— JOY UFEMA, RN, MS

---

apies such as massage may also prove beneficial in a comprehensive plan to manage depression.

Spiritual care

Each of the major standards-issuing agencies for end-of-life nursing practice has stipulated the need to attend to patients' spiritual concerns. (See *Spirituality in the scope of nursing practice.*) Performing this task well requires empathy, flexibility, and respect for the patient's and family's view of life and death—a view that may differ sharply from your own.

Defining spirituality

Part of the challenge of understanding spirituality as a concept lies in separating it from religion—both in your mind and in your patient care. For the purposes of this chapter, *spiritual* is defined as the aspect of a person that searches for meaning in life, as well as the aspect that connects person to person and person to nature, including animals. Spiritual care makes no assumptions about personal convictions and isn't necessarily religious. *Religion* is defined as that which connects a person with his idea of a

---

Spirituality in the scope of nursing practice

Major standards-issuing organizations all agree about the importance of spiritual care for patients at all stages in life, perhaps especially at the end of life. As a group, they make these assertions.

■ Spiritual assessment should, at minimum, determine the patient's religious affiliation, beliefs, and what spiritual practices he finds important.

■ Each patient should receive an individualized care plan that addresses physical, psychological, social, and spiritual needs to improve quality at the end of life.

■ Nurses should respect patients' religious and spiritual diversity with knowledge and sensitivity.

■ Spiritual and existential issues should be assessed and addressed systematically and skillfully.

Organizations that support and specify a spiritual component to nursing care include the American Association of Colleges of Nursing, American Nurses Association, Hospice and Palliative Nurses Association, Joint Commission on Accreditation of Healthcare Organizations, and National Consensus Project for Quality Palliative Care.

---

supreme being, a divine source, or a force that actively influences his life. Religion is a narrower concept than spirituality. Spiritual needs can be both religious and nonreligious.

Many people practice no specific religion, but they have a deep sense of a supreme being or power in their lives. How one defines a higher power is dependent on many beliefs and experiences. It's important to distinguish, early on, between a patient who practices no particular faith and a patient who has no belief in a divine source. The latter may call himself an atheist, nonbeliever, or skeptic. Asking a general question, such as, "What do you believe about life after death?" can help clarify if a patient has a faith-oriented spirituality.

For some people, religious faith and the support of a religious community bring comfort. Faith, at least theoretically, allows these patients and families to trust in God's love, wisdom, and care. Comfort comes from the notion that death is a temporary separation from loved ones who will be reunited in an afterlife where they will no longer experience pain or suffering.

At times, spiritual or religious beliefs can lead to distress and discomfort. People who fear judgment, punishment, and even eternal damnation may feel abandoned by God, their religious community, or both. While it's imperative that these patients be offered help from religious professionals, it's equally important that well-meaning family members and health professionals refrain from solving the patient's distress by advancing their own particular set of beliefs.

For many people, whether or not they practice a religion, a spiritual struggle arises at the end of life. There may be spiritual issues with finding purpose or forgiveness, saying goodbye, and coming to terms with beliefs about what transpires after death. For some, developing or enhancing an existing relationship with the transcendent may become more important. On the other hand, for those who don't believe in the power of the transcendent, it can be even more distressing when palliative care professionals make assumptions about the type of spiritual care that's helpful. No matter what spiritual conclusions a patient reaches, your goal is to support him in completing the psychological, social, and spiritual tasks of dying.

Assessment

During the initial assessment, you or the physician can talk to the patient about his wishes for spiritual and religious support. The answers you receive will vary widely between patients, including desires for specific rituals and practices before, during, and after death.

The first step in developing a plan of care is to determine if the patient belongs to a formal religion, has an informal set of beliefs, or has no sense of a supreme being or life after death. Thoroughly assess spiritual and religious preferences for both patient and family. Many families have a variety of religious and spiritual belief systems. You need not be expert in all of them, but you should become skillful in completing a spiritual assessment that will then form a plan of care to meet the patient's individual needs. There are a few commonly used spiritual assessment tools that can help you determine your patient's spiritual outlook.

Once you understand the patient's belief system, you can expand the assessment by asking simple questions about the rest of the family. For example, ask, "How does your belief system differ from your family's?" or, "How have your beliefs changed?"

Many patients experience some type of spiritual distress at the end of life. Often it's temporary. Signs and symptoms may include uncontrolled pain, irritability, depression, anxiety, anger, an inability to pray or participate in usual spiritual activities, or hopelessness. Addressing each of these issues in a holistic manner will help the patient become more comfortable. For example, investigate pain not just as a physical experience that warrants an increased drug dosage but also as a possible sign of unresolved psychosocial or spiritual issues; doing so will lead to more effective pain management. Identifying and addressing spiritual and other psychosocial problems will add valuable insight into an appropriate plan of care.

Continuum of spiritual interventions

Spiritual orientation	Interventions
Person to person, person to self	▪ Spending time with friends and family ▪ Writing letters ▪ Eating together ▪ Making videos or recordings for family ▪ Reviewing family photo albums ▪ Telling stories ▪ Facilitating forgiveness ▪ Making an ethical will ▪ Looking inward for strength
Person to nature	▪ Spending time outside or by a window ▪ Viewing pictures of the natural environment ▪ Keeping indoor plants
Person to animals	▪ Spending time with pets ▪ Viewing photos of animals
Informal beliefs about transcendence	▪ Saying prayers ▪ Practicing meditation ▪ Reading from spiritual or philosophical works ▪ Performing preferred rituals
Formal beliefs about transcendence	▪ Practicing religion ▪ Spending time with religious community ▪ Saying formalized prayers ▪ Making confession ▪ Performing religious rituals

Management

To address patients' spiritual issues, provide appropriate interventions along the continuum of spirituality. (See *Continuum of spiritual interventions.*) In a multicultural, multiethnic society, providing individualized spiritual care to each patient and family member can be one of the most challenging areas of palliative care. Support for patients and their family members' individual belief systems can be carried out with planning and coordination. The palliative plan of care should clearly identify the roles and expectations of every person supporting the patient, including representatives of various faiths.

The most basic level of spiritual care practice promotes a meaningful life. Practices that promote meaningful life include time alone, time with family, connection to nature, a calm environment, music, poetry, and art among other activities. Asking the patient about what gives his life meaning will direct caregivers in the most effective interventions. Participation in particular activities will vary with the patient's functional status. For example, a patient who enjoys writing poetry may replace that activity by listening to poetry if he becomes unable to write.

Ethical wills

Ethical wills are regaining popularity as a spiritual intervention in end-of-life care. They were first mentioned in the Bible. Ethical wills are a way for patients to share their values, express love and forgiveness, and offer valuable lessons to others. Patients can leave an ethical will by writing down important issues they experienced. The types of information contained in an ethical will can include the patient recounting important turning points in his life or how he faced challenges. Stories of important failures in life that led to personal development can also be very powerful. The patient may write the ethical will and choose to read it aloud at a special ceremony designed for this purpose. The patient could choose to leave the will to be read after his death, similar to a last will and testament. When the patient isn't near family and friends, a copy of the ethical will can be sent to those closest to him. Or the reading of the ethical will can be recorded and sent to family.

Cultural care

In the 2000 census of the United States, 65% of respondents identified themselves as White, 13% as Black, 13% as Hispanic, 4.5% as Asian–Pacific Islander, and 1.5% as American Indian/Alaskan. About 2.5% — a growing percentage — reported that they were bi-ethnic. As the population of the United States continues to diversify, nurses will need an increasing ability to develop rapport with ethnically varied patients and their families. Perhaps the most important requirement is a respect for and interest in your patients' cultural heritage. By developing an understanding of common cultural issues, you'll be better able to assist patients at the end of life. (See *Elements of cultural assessment*.)

You can open the door to a cultural exchange in many ways. For example, you might ask, "Some patients want to know all about their medical conditions, and others don't. What would you prefer?" Or you might ask, "Do you prefer to make your own medical decisions, or would you like someone else to make them for you?" To open the door further, ask, "Is there anything that would be helpful for us to know about your family, community, or religious or spiritual views about serious illness?"

Elements of cultural assessment

Every patient and family hold a unique set of beliefs that both adhere to and depart from the norms of their culture. To help understand their preferences, investigate points such as these:

- Implications of silence and eye contact
- Preferred form of address
- Effect of age and gender
- Permission to touch
- Acceptable modes of express-ing emotion
- Beliefs about what causes sick-ness and supports healing
- Importance of an individual versus a group
- Relationship between dis-cussing illness and causing illness
- Who may be present with the patient during death
- Methods of decision-making
- Definition of family
- Role of family in cultural life

- Dietary preferences and re-quirements
- Cultural rituals
- Coordination with culture-based healing techniques
- Interaction between spirituality and healing
- Importance of natural ele-ments
- Beliefs about God
- Concept of afterlife
- How and when the spirit leaves the body
- What makes life meaningful
- Preparation of the body
- Burial requirements
- Customs for mourning

If you can't understand the patient or the patient can't understand you, use an interpreter, possibly a family member, who can perform a word-for-word translation and also uphold the patient's confidentiality. When using an interpreter, look at the patient, not the translator, and speak directly to the patient. In other words, ask, "Where is your pain?" rather than "Would you ask him where his pain is?"

Particularly for end-of-life care, three important culturally influenced topics involve making decisions, talking about illness, and understanding advance directives. By working to understand your patients' cultural diversity, you can provide them with respectful care that meets their unique needs.

Making decisions

Medical care in the United States values autonomy; patients are empow-ered—indeed, expected—to make decisions about their health care. Other cultures have substantially different values. For example, cultures that value doing no harm over personal autonomy tend to prefer family-centered health care decisions and sometimes may make treatment decisions without the patient's input. In many societies, patients and families defer end-of-life decision-making to the physician, who is viewed as the expert. Some ethnic communities deem it appropriate to withhold potentially distressing information from mentally competent patients. Some cultures prefer to give the patient hope even during end-stage illness. Others view illness as a family event and not an individual event. Implicit in this culture is the concern about the impact of the person's death on the entire family. One of your most important cultural assessments involves understanding how your patient and his family prefer to make decisions.

Talking about illness

Health care professionals in the United States tend to value telling the "truth" about diagnoses and prognoses. In contrast, health care professionals in some cultures outside the United States may tend to conceal serious diagnoses from their patients. For example, when discussing cancer with patients or families, many African and Japanese physicians use terms such as "growth," "mass," "blood disease," or even "unclean tissue," to describe a disease. Chinese, Pakistani, and Hispanic community members are likely to protect terminally ill patients from the knowledge of their conditions.

Certain cultures perceive discussion of serious illness and death as disrespectful or impolite or feel that it may cause undue anxiety, depression, or loss of hope. Many also believe in the power of the spoken word and believe that discussion of illness or death may make it a reality. Members of these cultures may find a direct discussion of illness hurtful and harmful to health.

Along with the perspective of maintaining hope by not revealing terminal diagnoses is the notion that factors outside medical technology, such as divine intervention and personal coping mechanisms may play a more significant role in survival than medical intervention. To some patients and families, discussion of end-of-life care may be interpreted as lack of respect for the belief that one's fate is determined by God and not modern medicine.

Understanding advance directives

Many Americans of the prevailing White European culture have tried to establish and maintain some control over their last days by preparing advance directives. Members of other cultures and races may not be as likely to have an advance directive, for many reasons.

For one thing, a minority patient may not trust the faithful execution of the directive. For another, they may prefer to avoid the suggestion or admission of a terminal illness. These cultures may wish to protect patients from emotional and physical distress caused by directly addressing death and end-of-life care. Or they may feel that talking openly about a terminal illness will render the illness fatal.

Some cultures may prefer not to retain the autonomy that advance directives provide, believing instead that illness and death affect family and community. These patients may believe that coping with and making decisions about an end-stage illness shouldn't be left to the individual alone. Some patients may be reluctant to appoint one person as health care decision-maker because doing so may offend other members of the family, preferring instead to arrive at decisions by consensus.

Some cultures are more likely to view suffering as spiritually meaningful. Survival may be viewed as a demonstration of religious faith and life as always having some value. In other cultures, younger members are devoted to the reverent care of their elders and may opt for extraordinary measures to ensure life for as long as possible. In turn, ailing parents may consider it their responsibility to continue living for the emotional well-being of their adult children.

Cultural diversity

It's increasingly important for health care providers to solicit specific cultural information about different ethnic groups and their divergent backgrounds. (See *Cultural considerations*, pages 92 through 97.) Remember that most cultures share a respect for the elderly as well as for health care practitioners. In many cultures, refusal, opposition, even questioning may be considered rude. If we are to show compassion, we must think before we speak or act. This alone will go a long way toward bridging the gap in our diversities.

You can't possibly know all there is to know about every culture and religion, but you can and must be aware that there are other ways of looking at things besides your own. Listen and observe without being judgmental. Don't assume that your way of looking at things is the "right" way. Also, don't assume that a patient of a certain cultural background fits a stereotypical norm for that culture. Treat each patient and family as an individual unit with their own unique background and beliefs, doing your best to understand and interact with them on that level. As modern technology in medicine, communication, and education expands, we will be faced as never before with the challenge of providing care for all peoples. As spiritual beings, we can and should do so to the best of our abilities for the good of all life.

Cultural considerations

As a nurse, you typically interact with a diverse, multicultural population. Although negative stereotyping of different cultures must be avoided, it's nevertheless important to learn about the representative characteristics of different groups. Understanding various cultures will help you provide holistic interventions to meet the needs of the patient and family.

This table summarizes the health care beliefs and practices relating to dietary, communication, family roles, death rituals, health care practices and folk heath practices for five cultural groups that are common in the United States. Also summarized is the predominant Western Culture health care beliefs and practices.

Cultural group	Health care belief and illness philosophy
African Americans	■ May believe that illness is related to supernatural causes. ■ May seek advice and remedies from faith or folk healers. ■ May exhibit a stoic response to pain until it's unbearable and then seek emergency care. ■ Family oriented — customary for many family members to remain with a dying patient in the hospital. ■ May express grief by crying, screaming, praying, singing and reading scripture.
Arab Americans (Most trace their roots to Lebanon, Syria, Palestine, Egypt, and Iraq.)	■ Aura of silence surround some health problems such as sexually transmitted diseases, substance abuse, mental illness. ■ Devout Muslim may interpret illness as the will of Allah, a test of faith, representing a type of fatalistic view. ■ May rely on ritual cures or alternative therapies before seeing a health care provider. ■ Respect for the elderly — obliged to take care of their elderly relatives. ■ May express pain freely. ■ *Death:* Family or community members may want to prepare the body by washing and wrapping the body in unsewn white cloth. ■ Post-mortem examinations are discouraged unless required by law.

Dietary practices	Other considerations
■ May have food restrictions based on religious beliefs (such as not eating pork, if Muslim). ■ Have a higher occurrence of high blood pressure and obesity, which may be diet-related. ■ High occurrence of lactose intolerance with difficulty digesting milk and milk products. ■ May view cooked greens as good for health. ■ Traditional "soul" food diet is high in protein and fat.	■ *Values:* Family bonding, matriarchal, present orientation, spiritual orientation. ■ Tend to be affectionate, as shown by touching and hugging friends and loved ones. ■ Muslim women must keep their heads covered at all times. ■ *Primary religions:* Baptist, other Protestant denominations, Muslim.
■ Choose foods based on the humoral theory of balancing hot and cold. ■ Prefer dairy products, rice, and wheat breads. ■ May avoid pork and alcohol if Muslim. ■ Islam — observe month-long fast of Ramadan (begins about mid-October); those with chronic illness, pregnant, breast-feeding or menstruating women don't fast. ■ Don't mix milk and fish, sweet and sour, or hot and cold. ■ Don't use ice in drinks; believe that hot soup can help recovery.	■ *Values:* Family patriarchal and hierarchical, respect for elders, modesty, respectability and politeness. ■ Muslim women may avoid eye contact as a show of modesty. ■ Many Muslim women wear the traditional hijab (head cover). ■ Respect for higher education and advanced degrees. ■ Use same-sex family members as interpreters. ■ Preventive care among adults is not highly valued. ■ *Primary religions:* Muslim (Islam), Protestant, Greek Orthodox and Catholic.

(continued)

Cultural considerations *(continued)*

Cultural group	Health care belief and illness philosophy
Asian Americans (Includes Cambodians, Chinese, Filipino, Indian, Indonesian, Korean, Pakistani, Thai, Vietnamese.)	■ Asian Americans have differing health views depending on their particular subculture. *Chinese:* may believe illness results when a person fails to act in harmony with nature, such as yin and yang. *Filipino:* may believe dying is God's plan and that neither the patient nor the health care provider should interfere with God's will. *Korean:* may adhere to traditional values that dictate that patient should die at home. *Japanese:* May believe that illness is karma, resulting from behavior in the current life or a past life. ■ May value ability to endure pain and grief with silent stoicism . ■ Typically very family oriented; extended family should be involved in care of dying patient.
Latino Americans (Includes Caribbean, Mexico, Central and South America populations.)	■ May view illness as a sign of weakness, punishment for evil or retribution for shameful behavior. ■ May use the terms "hot" and "cold in reference to vital elements needed to restore equilibrium to the body. ■ May consult with a curandero (healer) or voodoo priest (Caribbean). ■ May view pain as a necessary part of life and believe that enduring pain is a sign of strength (especially men). ■ May have open expression of grief, such as praying for the dead, saying the rosary. ■ May use various amulets to protect individual from evil. ■ The family members are typically involved in all aspects of decision-making such as terminal illness.
Native Americans	■ May turn to a medicine man to determine the true cause of an illness, such as why a person is out of harmony with nature. ■ May value the ability to endure pain or grief with silent stoicism. ■ Views death as part of life cycle.

Dietary practices	Other considerations
■ Hot/cold theory (ying and yang) often involved. Example: curing a "hot" disease such as arthritis may require cold foods or medicines. ■ Hindu religious food practices: Many refrain from eating cows, some are lacto-vegetarians eating only milk products and vegetables. ■ Eat rice with most meals; may use chopsticks. ■ *Chinese:* may use herbalist or acupuncturists before seeking medical help. ■ Sodium intake is typically high (salting and drying foods and use of condiments).	■ *Values:* Group orientation, submission to authority, respect for elders, respect for past, modesty, conformity, tradition. ■ May believe that prolonged eye contact is rude and invasion of privacy. ■ Tend to be very modest; prefer same-sex clinicians. ■ May nod without necessarily understanding (especially elderly Japanese patients). ■ May prefer to maintain a comfortable physical distance between the patient and the health care provider. ■ *Primary religions:* Buddhist, Protestant, Catholic, Shinto (Japanese), Hindu and Islam (India), Taoism, Zen Buddhism, Confucianism.
■ May use herbal teas and soup to aid in recuperation. ■ The traditional diet is basically vegetarian with an emphasis on corn, corn products, beans, rice, and breads. ■ Select beans and tortillas are staples and may be eaten at every meal. ■ Typically eat a lot of fresh fruits and vegetables, however, variety in diet may be limited. ■ High occurrence of obesity, particularly central obesity, that raises the risk of diabetes and heart disease.	■ *Values:* Group emphasis, extended family, fatalism, present orientation. ■ May have fatalistic view of life. ■ May see no reason to submit to mammograms or vaccinations. ■ May need private room where grief can be expressed openly. ■ May be modest (especially women). ■ Use same-sex family members as interpreters. ■ *Primary religion:* Roman Catholic.
■ Diet may be deficient in vitamin D because many suffer from lactose intolerance or don't drink milk. ■ Obesity and diabetes are major health concerns.	■ *Values:* Bonding to family or group, sharing with others, present orientation, extended family, cooperation with and acceptance of nature.

(continued)

Cultural considerations *(continued)*

Cultural group	Health care belief and illness philosophy
Native Americans *(continued)*	■ Burial practices vary among tribal groups. Example: Navajos fear death and distance themselves from death. ■ May avoid touching the dead or dying person. ■ Many believe that the spirit of a dying person cannot leave the body until the family is there. ■ Grief tends to be family oriented with all members assuming roles in the grieving process.
Western Culture (The Western health care system is a subculture of white Western culture of European roots.)	■ Members of this culture value technology almost exclusively in the struggle to conquer disease. ■ The strong shared belief in the biomedical approach may result in serious barriers to communication with other cultures who choose to use alternative or complementary therapies. ■ Health is generally understood to be the absence, minimization, or control of disease. ■ Hospitalization may foster an atmosphere that requires the patient or family to be compliant, dependent, and vulnerable to get needs met. ■ Health care emphasis is shifting from treating diseases to disease prevention and health promotion.

Dietary practices	Other considerations
■ Herbs are used in the treatment of many illnesses to cleanse the body of ill spirits or poisons.	■ May divert their eyes to the floor when they are praying or paying attention. ■ Raised to be reserved and non-committal, may respond to assessment questions with silence or monosyllables. ■ *Belief system:* Characterized by intense relationship with nature.
■ Health care facilities often have standard dietary guidelines, which may or may not consider cultural variations. ■ Eating utensils consist mainly of knife, fork and spoon. ■ Three meals eaten daily is typical. ■ American culture values convenience and may substitute ready-to-eat (fast food) items typically low in nutrition. ■ Eating out is a growing American cultural trend. Meals eaten out tend to be higher in calories, fat, and sodium . ■ Growing occurrence of obesity.	■ *Values:* Independence, self reliance and individualism, resistance to authority, nuclear or blended family, innovation, emphasis on youth, future orientation, competition. ■ Health care is a culture of its own rituals and language often incomprehensible to patients and families of other cultures.

8 Patients with cancer

Cancer is the second leading cause of death in the United States and the most common diagnosis in palliative and hospice care. The latter fact probably stems from several characteristics particular to cancer. For one thing, it's possible to predict the course of most forms of cancer relatively accurately, which gives physicians some confidence in making referrals to end-of-life care. For another, end-stage cancer typically causes symptoms that can be relieved.

Lung, breast, prostate, and colon cancers cause most cancer deaths. Prostate cancer, the main hormone-related cancer in men, claims 30,000 lives yearly. Breast cancer kills 40,000 women yearly. Colon cancer kills 64,000 men and women yearly. And lung cancer, the leading cause of cancer deaths among Americans, kills 163,000 people yearly.

Often, it's metastasis that causes the patient's death, not the primary disease. Breast and prostate cancers typically metastasize to the brain, bone, lung, and liver. Advanced non–small-cell lung cancer (the most common lung cancer in hospice) typically spreads to structures around the lungs, such as the chest wall, heart, blood vessels, trachea, and esophagus. Colon cancer metastasizes to the lungs and liver.

The symptoms of end-stage cancer correspond to its spread. If a breast cancer patient has lung metastasis, for example, she'll most likely have dyspnea. If cancer has spread to the liver, she probably will have anorexia. If the cancer is in the bone, she may have a pathologic fracture. Any of these metastases may cause pain.

Despite the common belief that cancer deaths are excruciatingly painful, virtually all pain in dying cancer patients can be relieved. In fact, virtually all end-stage cancer symptoms can be effectively reduced and managed. What's more, patients dying of cancer typically have time to make apologies, ask forgiveness, give forgiveness, and say "I love you" and "Good-bye." By managing the symptoms common to end-stage cancer—such as pain, dyspnea, dehydration and anorexia, nausea and vomiting, fatigue, sleep problems, and emergencies—you can help make the patient's final days among his most meaningful.

Pain

Nearly everyone who's diagnosed with cancer expects to have pain —particularly if the cancer can't be cured. Many patients believe the closer they get to death the more unbearable their pain will be. It's true that cancer, especially end-stage cancer, can be painful. As tumors grow, they press on nearby tissues or infiltrate other organs. However, it's also true that cancer pain can be relieved in nearly all dying patients. Here's what you need to know about pain and ways to relieve it for patients at the end of life.

Types of cancer pain

A growing tumor causes a series of exchanges between peripheral nerves, spinal cord, and brain. Nociceptors, nerve cells that sense the presence of harm, transmit signals from the nerves to the spinal cord. There they interact with specialized nerve cells that act as gatekeepers, filtering the pain messages on their way to the brain. In severe pain, the "gates" are wide open and the message travels quickly to the brain, while milder pain travels at a slower speed.

Once the pain message reaches the brain, it's interpreted as a physical sensation with complex links to both emotions and thought processes. Individual differences in the number of nociceptors, spinal cord gates, or cells in the nervous systems can cause differences in how much pain a patient experiences. So does culture. Culture not only determines how patients react to pain (crying loudly versus quiet stoicism); it also plays a role in determining how patients perceive pain.

The location and type of pain in end-stage cancer patients play a role in its sensation as well.

Somatic pain
Somatic pain occurs in skeletal tissue, muscles, and the surface of the skin. Patients usually describe somatic pain as dull or aching but localized; pain from bone metastases is somatic. Somatic pain responds well to most analgesics.

Visceral pain

Visceral pain results from infiltration, compression, extension, or stretching of the chest, abdominal, or pelvic viscera. Pain from pancreatic cancer is visceral. Patients usually describe visceral pain as pressure, as deep pain, or as squeezing pain. Visceral pain usually is diffuse and not well localized.

Neuropathic pain

This type of pain develops when a tumor presses on nerves or the spinal cord or when cancer spreads inside the spinal cord. Patients with neuropathic pain say it feels like burning or tingling. It may be localized to a specific spot, or it may be diffuse, affecting large or patchy areas.

Wind-up pain

When nerves transmit pain impulses to the brain for long periods of time, they become more effective at sending pain signals, and the brain becomes more effective at recognizing them. This heightened signaling causes wind-up pain, a type of pain that continues to intensify, becoming more difficult to treat the longer it continues.

Assessment

You can't know how much pain a patient is having unless you ask. Then you have to believe the answer. This simple concept ensures that patients with end-stage cancer receive exemplary pain relief.

Instead of relying on facial grimacing, blood pressure readings, or sleep status, just ask the patient how much he hurts. Instead of assuming that patients tend to overestimate or underestimate their pain, simply accept that the true gauge of patient pain is the patient.

Tools

The most effective way to gauge your patient's pain and how it changes over time is to use a pain rating scale. (See *Pain assessment tools.*) Choose the most appropriate of the many such scales that are available, including these:

■ a numbered scale from 0 (no pain) to 10 (worst pain possible)
■ a series of faces with increasing emotions, a happy face indicating no pain and increasingly distressed faces for increasing pain
■ a visual analog scale, which uses a straight line, with the far left side meaning no pain and the far right side meaning the worst pain imaginable
■ a categorical scale, with four categories to describe pain (none [0], mild [1–3], moderate [4–8], severe [7–10])
■ a word scale using verbal descriptions of pain (horrible, burning, excruciating, agonizing, aching, and so on)

Pain assessment tools

Numeric pain rating scale
A numeric rating scale can help the patient quantify his pain. Have him choose a number from 0 (indicating no pain) to 10 (indicating the worst pain imaginable) to reflect his current pain level. He can either circle the number on the scale itself or verbally state the number that best describes his pain.

No pain	0	1	2	3	4	5	6	7	8	9	10	Pain as bad as it can be

Visual analog scale
To use the visual analog scale, ask the patient to place a mark on the scale to indicate his current level of pain.

No pain |————————————————————————| Pain as bad as it can be

Wong-Baker FACES pain rating scale
A child or an adult with language difficulties may not be able to describe in words or numbers the pain he's feeling. If so, try a pain rating scale that uses facial expressions to gauge his pain level. Ask the patient to choose the face that best represents the severity of his pain. Explain the faces using a 0-to-10 scale and the descriptions included on the tool.

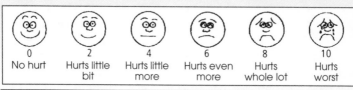

| 0 | 2 | 4 | 6 | 8 | 10 |
| No hurt | Hurts little bit | Hurts little more | Hurts even more | Hurts whole lot | Hurts worst |

From Hockenberry MJ, Wilson D, Winkelstein ML: *Wong's Essentials of Pediatric Nursing,* ed. 7, St. Louis, 2005, p.1259. Used with permission. Copyright, Mosby.

■ colors on a spectrum, starting on the left with an icy white-blue and ending with a deep red on the right. This scale is more prone to misinterpretation than the others because some patients may perceive icy-blue as a more painful color than deep red.

Questions
Also, ask your patient to describe the details of his pain using such questions as these:

Describing the pain

If a patient has trouble pinpointing the character of his pain in his own words, you can help by providing descriptive words he can choose from. Offer the choices in small, related groups, such as, "Is your pain aching, burning, or stabbing?" Here are some descriptive words to get you started.

- Aching
- Burning
- Constant
- Crushing
- Dull
- Electric
- Gnawing

- Heavy
- Intermittent
- Pins and needles
- Pressing
- Prickling
- Pulsing
- Searing

- Sharp
- Shooting
- Spasm
- Stabbing
- Throbbing

- Can you describe your pain? (See *Describing the pain*.)
- Where does it hurt?
- Does it always hurt? Are there times your pain is better? Worse?
- What else can you tell me about your pain?
- What do you want your pain medication to do?

As your patient nears death, he'll sleep more and wake less; eventually, he'll become unresponsive. Most patients at the end of life can no longer tell you how much or what kind of pain they're having. What's more, nonverbal cues—such as changes in vital signs, moaning, grimacing, and sleep status—aren't reliable indicators of pain in a dying patient. Don't be fooled into thinking that a patient has no pain just because he can't describe it. Keep giving the same analgesics, at the same dosage and on the same schedule that the patient was receiving them before he became nonverbal. Keep giving them until the patient dies. If needed, change from the oral to the rectal route; many analgesics, including morphine, controlled-release opioids, and nonsteroidal anti-inflammatory drugs (NSAIDs) are absorbed well from the rectum.

Management

The number one goal in caring for dying patients with pain is to remove the obstacles to relieving your patient's pain, including the errant beliefs of health care providers, patients, families, and administrators. (See *Sources of ineffective pain management*.)

Sources of ineffective pain management

Despite compelling, long-standing evidence for the importance of aggressive pain management, too many patients are living and dying with too much pain. Here are some reasons why pain management tends to be ineffective.

Sources	Reasons
Physicians and nurses	■ Inadequate knowledge of pain management principles ■ Reluctance to accept that pain really is what the patient says it is ■ Fear of opioids ■ Assumption that pain in dying people sometimes can't be relieved ■ Inadequate time
Patients and families	■ Fear of opioids ■ Fear of being labeled a bad patient ■ Fear of addiction ■ Fatalism that pain is part of dying
Health care systems and facilities	■ Concerns about regulatory scrutiny ■ Insufficient knowledge about opioid use ■ Reluctance to accept the expertise and skill of hospice nurses and physicians ■ Costs

Principles of pain management

Many people fear pain management almost as much as they fear pain itself; to help provide your dying patient with the pain relief he needs and deserves, keep these points in mind.

■ Pain is whatever the patient says it is.

■ Pain can be relieved in virtually all patients at the end of life.

■ Treatment of a dying patient's pain shouldn't be withheld while the cause is determined.

■ Assess and reassess the patient's pain continually.

■ Use standardized pain assessment tools.

■ If the gut works, use it. The oral route is the preferred route.

■ For most patients receiving end-of-life care, analgesics should be given on a schedule around the clock, not "as necessary."

■ Make sure the patient has analgesic doses available for breakthrough pain—in the same drug he's receiving for around-the-clock pain control.

■ There's no "ceiling" dose of opioids in a patient with end-stage cancer.
■ Anticipate adverse effects, and treat them before they arise.
■ Use adjunct drugs as needed according to the patient's symptoms
■ Include meditation, music, and other nondrug interventions in the plan of care to relieve pain. (See *Nondrug interventions for pain.*)
■ Provide ongoing instruction in pain management to the patient and family.

 ALERT Escalating intractable pain is a medical emergency that requires prompt attention. Stay in contact with the patient's physician until the pain is relieved. The patient may need surgery, radiation, or sedation. If the patient is at home, a short-term inpatient stay for pain management may be warranted.

Steps of pain management
Whether a patient with end-stage cancer has moderate or severe pain, the best course is to maintain a steady drug level in his blood by giving analgesics around the clock. To avoid sleep interruptions, the patient may want to double the dose taken closest to bedtime. Here's a common stepped approach for keeping the pain in check.

Step 1 For patients with mild to moderate pain (pain rating from 1 to 3) a nonopioid drug such as those listed here is the best choice. Mild pain should be relieved within 12 hours.
■ *acetaminophen:* suppositories, tablets, capsules, gel-caps, or oral solution
■ *aspirin:* tablets or suppositories
■ *ibuprofen or other NSAID:* tablets, capsules, or suspension

Step 2 If the pain persists or increases (pain rating from 4 to 6), add a mild opioid to acetaminophen or an NSAID. Moderate pain should be relieved within 8 hours.
■ *Combunox (ibuprofen/oxycodone):* tablets
■ *Darvocet or Trycet (acetaminophen/propoxyphene):* tablets
■ *Darvon (propoxyphene):* tablets, capsules
■ *Darvon compound (aspirin/propoxyphene/caffeine):* pulvules
■ *Lortab or Vicodin (aspirin/codeine):* tablets, capsules, oral solution, elixir, caplets
■ *Percocet or Roxicet (acetaminophen/oxycodone):* tablets, capsules, caplets, oral solution
■ *Percodan or Roxiprin (aspirin/oxycodone):* tablets
■ *Tylenol #2, #3, or #4 (acetaminophen/codeine):* tablets, oral solution, suspension, elixir
■ *Ultram (tramadol):* tablets
■ *Vicoprofen (ibuprofen/hydrocodone):* tablets

Nondrug interventions for pain

Sometimes a simple position change or back rub is all that's needed to reduce pain. These comfort measures can also increase the effectivenesss of analgesics. Other nondrug measures include:

- Acupressure
- Acupuncture
- Aromatherapy
- Gentle massage
- Humor
- Music
- Pets

- Prayer and meditation
- Propping painful legs or arms on pillows
- Therapeutic touch
- Use of a heating pad, ice pack, or both

Because acetaminophen can cause liver damage or failure, especially in patients who consume alcohol, don't give more than 4 grams (4,000 mg) daily. If the patient takes an analgesic that contains aspirin, make sure to assess him for stomach upset and increased bleeding.

Step 3 If pain is severe (pain rating from 7 to 10), the patient will need a stronger opioid, such as those listed here. Start with a short-acting form. Severe pain should be relieved within 4 hours.
- *hydromorphone:* tablets, extended-release capsules, oral solution, suppositories; I.M., I.V. or subcutaneous injection; I.M., I.V., or subcutaneous high-potency injection
- *morphine sulfate:* tablets; extended-release tablets; controlled-release tablets; sustained-release capsules; oral solution; concentrated oral solution; suppositories; I.M., I.V., or subcutaneous injection; extended-release epidural injection; epidural and intrathecal injection
- *oxycodone:* immediate-release capsules and tablets, controlled-release tablets, oral solution, concentrated oral solution

For breakthrough pain, each dose should be 10% to 15% of the total daily dose. Usually, doses are ordered q 1 hour, p.r.n. Here are some examples of doses designed for breakthrough pain:
- morphine 5 mg q 4 hours P.O. around-the-clock with 5 mg q 1 hour P.O. p.r.n. for breakthrough pain
- oxycodone 5 mg q 4 hours P.O. around-the-clock with 5 mg q 1 hour P.O. p.r.n. for breakthrough pain.
- hydromorphone 1 mg q 4 hours P.O. around-the-clock regularly with 0.5 to 1 mg q 1 hour P.O. p.r.n. for breakthrough pain.

ALERT Meperidine (Demerol) produces a metabolite that's toxic to the nervous system. Don't give it to patients with end-stage cancer or other patients in end-of-life care.

Fentanyl (Duragesic) is another commonly used opioid for chronic pain because of its ease of use (transdermal patch) and the long period between doses (usually 72 hours). If the patient currently receives morphine and you need to switch to fentanyl, use an equianalgesic scale to establish the correct dosage. (See *Converting to fentanyl.*)

To determine the patient's total morphine dose, you'll have to include both the doses he receives around the clock and the doses he receives for breakthrough pain. In other words, if the patient takes morphine 60 mg P.O. q 4 hours plus one 30-mg breakthrough dose in 24 hours, perform this computation:

60 mg $\times$ 6 = 360 mg + 30 mg = 390 mg total morphine in 24 hours.

Then, using an equianalgesic chart, you'll see that he can switch to a 100-mcg fentanyl patch. Keep in mind, however, that because the equianalgesic chart covers wide ranges of morphine doses per fentanyl dose, some hospice agencies use a more specific conversion ratio. Here's how to do it:

First, determine the fentanyl dose by dividing the morphine dose by 100 using the ratio method below.

100 : 1 :: 390 : x. Solving for x, the result is 39 mg.

Now, convert milligrams to micrograms: 39 $\times$ 100 = 3,900 mcg.

Divide that by 24: 3,900/24 = 162.5 mcg fentanyl.

Using this formula, the patient should be using either a 150-mcg or a 175-mcg fentanyl patch, depending on the pain assessment.

Adverse effects

Although morphine is the drug closest to our body's own natural pain-killers, it isn't without adverse effects. All opioids share these common secondary reactions. Watch for and be prepared to treat these reactions.

Constipation   Morphine almost always causes constipation; start treating it as soon as morphine therapy starts. Giving a stool softener and fiber laxative once or twice daily may be sufficient if the patient still has reasonable food and fluid intake. Stronger preparations such as lactulose (Chronolac) may be needed and can be adjusted easily to the patient's bowel status. Some patients need a regular regimen of oral laxatives plus a periodic rectal preparation, such as bisacodyl suppository.

Sleepiness   Usually, sleepiness goes away as the patient's body grows accustomed to the dosage. It may recur temporarily at each dosage increase. If it persists, the morphine may not be causing it. Instead, the patient may have ongoing drowsiness from progression of the illness itself. (See *A time to listen,* page 108.)

Converting to fentanyl

If you're converting a patient from morphine to fentanyl, use this equianalgesic scale to help you make the switch. Don't forget that the morphine dose is in milligrams and the fentanyl dose is in micrograms.

Morphine (mg)	Fentanyl (mcg)	Morphine (mg)	Fentanyl (mcg)
60–134	25	585–674	175
135–224	50	675–764	200
225–314	75	765–854	225
315–404	100	855–944	250
405–494	125	945–1,034	275
495–584	150	1035–1,124	300

Nausea Morphine causes nausea in a substantial percentage of people. It can be prevented with prochlorperazine (Compazine) given for the first 3 to 4 days of morphine therapy. Hospice patients who are easily nauseated or continuously feel a little sick to their stomach should be started on metoclopramide (Reglan) right away.

Itching Itchiness can be treated with diphenhydramine (Benadryl) but this drug also causes drowsiness. An alternative option may be loratadine (Claritin). Frequent application of lotion to the skin or applying cool-water compresses can also be helpful.

Dry mouth Try relieving the patient's dry mouth with small sips of water, ice chips, peppermint candies, and frequent mouth care. If these interventions aren't sufficient, he may need a saliva substitute.

Morphine misconceptions
Patients who became itchy or nauseated when they received morphine in the past may have been told that these symptoms meant they were allergic to morphine. This is a fairly common nursing error. Nausea, itchiness, and sleepiness are not allergic reactions. They are self-limiting effects that may be distressing but are easily treated. True morphine allergies are rare.

Sometimes morphine or other opioids are blamed for causing confusion and hallucinations when these symptoms actually are caused by imminent death. People who are near death may appear confused and disoriented;

EXPERT INSIGHTS

A time to listen

I work the evening shift at an extended-care facility. Recently, a dying patient's two adult children asked the staff to "lighten up" on their father's pain medication so he could talk with them one last time. How would you respond to such a request? — P.A., Minn.

Let me answer by telling you about an experience I had with a patient who was dying from ovarian cancer with metastasis to her bowel. She'd been in pain and restless until we began giving morphine sulfate (Roxanol). Her devoted daughters remained at her bedside day and night, bathing and repositioning her and offering her tiny sips of tea. They adored their mother and lived to hear the two or three sentences she'd utter every 24 hours.

One night I stopped in her room to check on her condition and provide support. Afterward, the two daughters followed me out into the hall.

"We want you to stop giving the Roxanol, please," said one. "Mother is too sleepy to talk."

"I'm concerned that if we do that your dear mother will be in pain again," I replied.

"Well, we need to hear her talk. She hasn't talked all night or all day."

"That's because she's too weak from the cancer," I said. "I think she's going to die soon."

The daughters gasped in unison as if I'd just delivered a new diagnosis. "But we need to hear her talk!"

"I'm so sorry. But even if we stop the Roxanol, your mother won't be able to talk. She's dying now. I think she can hear you but she's too tired to reply. She really does need this good pain medicine. But she also needs to hear you tell her how much you love her and that you're going to stay with her."

After we hugged, they went back into their mother's room. I watched as they sat on either side of their mother and talked gently about their love for her.

Now it was her turn to listen.

— JOY UFEMA, RN, MS

they commonly speak to unseen people. Most patients seem more at ease and peaceful after having this experience. However, normally alert and oriented patients who are still caring for themselves may also experience these effects. Sometimes the side effects are mild and the patient can learn to ignore them. In other patients, these changes are very bothersome and different opioids or non-traditional options, such as an anticonvulsant, should be tried. In patients who have severe reactions to morphine and other opioids, trials of I.V. lidocaine have been used successfully.

Dyspnea

In end-stage cancer, dyspnea is a common symptom. It may stem from several sources. Tumors growing in the lung take up space and reduce the space available for air. If the tumor presses against the bronchi or invades bronchial structures, the airways become narrowed, making the work of breathing more difficult. Damage to pulmonary tissues from radiation treatments may cause dyspnea as well.

If the patient's abdomen or liver is enlarged, the diaphragm may be pushed up against the lungs. Reduced lung volume means increased dyspnea. Likewise if the patient has ascites or a severe bowel obstruction.

Pneumonia is another common cause of dyspnea in dying cancer patients. So are sepsis and other infections. Fear, loneliness, guilt, and anxiety are common feelings in patients with end-stage cancer. These emotional states commonly cause feelings of breathlessness in dying patients as well.

Assessment

You can't know how much dyspnea a patient is having simply by counting respirations or auscultating lung sounds. Just as with pain, you must go to the source and ask your patients how hard it is for them to breathe. This may be especially important for terminally ill cancer patients with dyspnea. While patients with end-stage emphysema are often experts in understanding and managing their breathlessness, patients with primary lung cancer or metastatic disease may never have experienced ongoing or severe shortness of breath. They need much support and reassurance in addition to superlative care. A complete assessment is the crucial first step in helping dyspneic dying patients breathe easier.

Tools

You can use pain assessment tools to measure a patient's dyspnea as well. For instance, a visual analog scale is simply a flat line, most often horizontal and 10 centimeters long. By making one diagonal slash along the line, the patient can rate how hard it is for him to breathe. The left end of the line means no dyspnea; the right end of the line means the worst dyspnea ever.

A numerical rating scale, also the same as the one used for pain, places an actual value on the patient's dyspnea, with 0 meaning no dyspnea and 10 meaning the worst dyspnea imaginable. Ask the patient to choose a number based on how hard it is to breathe. If the patient can conceptualize adequately, you won't need a visual aid. Simply ask him, "On a scale from zero to ten, with zero meaning no shortness of breath and ten meaning the most out of breath you can imagine, what number would you use to rate your breathlessness right now?"

You can also use a series of facial expressions or a list of descriptive words to help the patient rate his level of dyspnea. If you print the words on paper, the patient can simply circle or make a mark to choose the word he wants. You also may consider using colors on a spectrum to help the patient rate his dyspnea, but keep in mind that this system may be more easy to misinterpret than the others.

Also keep in mind that many patients with end-stage cancer and dyspnea may not like using these rating tools. If they've had dyspnea for a long time, they may find the tools a waste of energy, especially if you try a new one with a patient who's used to using something else.

Observations
Use observations to augment the patient's report or if the patient can't speak or is too tired or short of breath to rate his breathlessness. Objective dyspnea assessments include:
- deep, sighing respirations
- frequent position changes
- grimacing
- grunting
- labored breathing
- moaning
- pushing others away
- rapid breathing
- reaching out with hands and arms
- restlessness
- shallow breathing
- tactile defensiveness (dislike of being touched).

Auscultation
Certainly, it's valuable to listen to a patient's lung fields as he breathes. However, for a breathless patient with end-stage cancer, remember that this assessment may take substantial energy reserves from the patient. When a patient is dying of end-stage lung cancer or has significant pulmonary

metastases, the truth is that little can be gained by listening to his lungs. The wheezes, stridor, rales, and rhonchi will remain and most likely increase. Absent lung sounds from removal of a lung or lobe will not reappear. Treatments to reduce dyspnea in end-of-life settings are provided according to how the patient feels, not the amount of crackles you hear in his lung bases.

Management

The most common and effective interventions for patients with end-stage cancer and dyspnea are oxygen therapy, drug therapy, environmental changes, and repositioning.

Oxygen

Oxygen therapy is a simple and effective treatment. It reduces dyspnea in end-stage cancer patients by increasing oxygen saturation while decreasing airway resistance and the work of breathing. Even if the patient's blood gas levels are adequate, the simple flow of air over the nasal mucosa often helps dying patients feel like they're breathing easier.

The two usual means of oxygen delivery, a nasal cannula or mask, can be used interchangeably in end-of-life settings. Patients who need a high flow of oxygen typically need it by mask; however, some end-stage cancer patients feel claustrophobic under the mask and prefer a cannula. Some patients who use a cannula during the day prefer a mask at night or when their noses are irritated or clogged.

Sometimes patients with end-stage cancer or their families believe that the need for supplemental oxygen means that death is near. They also might believe that once oxygen has started, the patient will die if the cannula or mask is removed. Provide calm teaching and support to help patients and families understand that oxygen therapy is a tool to promote comfort and that the patient's illness will continue to progress with or without oxygen therapy in place. If the patient becomes irritated by the cannula or mask and continually tries to remove it, help the family accept the patient's wishes rather than aggravating the patient by continuing to place the device back on his face.

Drug therapy

Whether a dyspneic end-stage cancer patient is at home or in a hospital, long-term care facility, palliative care unit, or any other type of end-of-life care setting, the same general rule applies. When it comes to drug therapy, if the gut works, use it.

Morphine Opioids such as oxycodone, fentanyl, and methadone all relieve dyspnea, but morphine is the most used and best studied of the opioids.

Usually, it takes less morphine to relieve dyspnea than it does to relieve pain. In patients who aren't already taking morphine for pain relief, start with a fairly low dose and increase it slowly.

Liquid morphine is especially simple to give, easily adjusted, and reduces both cough and dyspnea. It can be given by schedule or as needed. Breakthrough doses can be given if dyspnea increases before the next scheduled dose.

In general, nebulized morphine probably has no benefit over an oral form in reducing dyspnea. Patients dying from chronic obstructive pulmonary disease (COPD) or other chronic breathing disorders may respond better to nebulized morphine than patients with end-stage cancer.

As with morphine given to relieve pain, morphine given to reduce dyspnea has adverse effects. Prevent them when possible, treat them when needed, and help patients and their families understand which effects are usually temporary. When patients and their families understand how morphine will help, symptom management is more effective.

 ALERT Nausea and itching can and should be treated even though these symptoms are temporary. Many patients who vomit after taking their first dose of morphine or are kept awake all night with unrelenting itching refuse to take any more morphine, and no patient dying of end-stage cancer should have to choose between nausea and dyspnea. By anticipating these adverse effects, preventing them when possible, treating them effectively, and teaching patients and families what to expect, you can increase your ability to use morphine successfully to reduce dyspnea.

Although extremely rare in hospice patients, morphine can cause the release of histamines. When histamine contracts the smooth muscles in the walls of the lungs and blood vessels, increased dyspnea, wheezing, and thick, sticky mucus may result.

Corticosteroids Given by mouth or inhaler, these drugs reduce airway inflammation. The many adverse effects that occur with long-term use of corticosteroids typically don't cause problems for patients with end-stage cancer. These drugs can be very useful in patients with underlying COPD or asthma.

Anxiolytics Most strong emotions will increase respirations, and many can make breathing difficult. End-stage cancer patients with dyspnea often feel panicky, and anxiolytics can be very helpful. Keep in mind, however, that they won't do much to reduce dyspnea unrelated to panic and anxiety.

The benzodiazepines alprazolam (Xanax), lorazepam (Ativan), and diazepam (Valium) are the most commonly used and the most effective. Longer-acting benzodiazepines (such as Xanax XR) may be used for chronic dyspnea. Always start with a small dose and increase slowly.

Other drugs Other drugs may help reduce dyspnea as well, depending on its cause.

Angiotensin-converting enzyme (ACE) inhibitors, such as enalapril (Vasotec), ramipril (Altace), captopril (Capoten), and benazepril (Lotensin), prevent worsening of heart function and lighten the heart's workload. Watch for light-headedness and a persistent, dry cough.

Diuretics, such as furosemide (Lasix), bumetanide (Bumex), and triam-terene (Dyrenium), eliminate excess fluid, thereby reducing the work of the heart and lungs, making breathing easier.

Beta blockers, such as bisoprolol (Zebeta), extended-release metoprolol (Toprol XL) and carvedilol (Coreg), decrease the heart's need for blood and oxygen by reducing its workload. They also help the heart beat more regularly.

Digoxin, a cardiac glycoside, helps the heart beat more strongly and effectively, possibly reducing dyspnea. Watch for digoxin toxicity, confusion, nausea, and visual disturbances. These may result from changes in the dying patient's metabolism and kidney function.

Vasodilators, such as hydralazine (Apresoline), isosorbide dinitrate (Isordil, Sorbitrate), and nitroglycerin, expand the blood vessels, lowering cardiac resistance. Watch for headaches and dizziness.

Bronchodilators open the airways by relaxing the surrounding muscles. Beta$_2$ agonists usually are inhaled and include short-acting drugs whose effects last from 3 to 6 hours; use these drugs only when the patient needs immediate relief.

Environmental interventions

Changing the air around a dyspneic patient is a simple and important intervention to help breathing feel easier. Open the windows. Turn on the air conditioning. Use a fan to stir the air and provide a direct, gentle breeze.

Also, dress the patient in loose clothing. Keep the surrounding area uncluttered. And try applying cool cloths to the patient's forehead or the back of his neck.

If appropriate to the particular patient, suggest prayer or meditation to reduce breathlessness. Playing soft music or the television can provide diversion. Teaching breathing techniques and chest relaxation is another powerful way to help end-stage cancer patients breathe easier. (See *Teaching patients to decrease dyspnea*, pages 114 and 115.)

Repositioning

Sometimes the simplest acts provide the most relief. Helping a breathless dying patient change position is sometimes all that's needed. With enough pillows, even the weakest dyspneic patient can be supported in an upright position. Comfortable specialty pillows are available as well. Reading pil-

COMFORT & CARE

Teaching patients to decrease dyspnea

Here are six tools you can teach to help your patient ease the discomfort of dyspnea. Some patients like to stick with one technique; others prefer to choose among several when they feel overwhelmed by breathlessness.

Technique	Instructions
Pursed-lip breathing	■ Relax. Let your neck and shoulders droop. ■ Breathe in slowly. ■ Purse your lips like you're going to whistle, and blow out slowly and evenly while keeping your lips pursed. ■ Try to take at least twice as long to blow out as you did to breathe in. ■ Keep this up until you feel less breathless. ■ Use pursed-lip breathing whenever you do anything that makes you short of breath, such as walking or climbing stairs.
Forward slump	■ This forward position gives your lungs a little more room in your chest. ■ Sit in a comfortable chair with your feet spread about shoulder width apart. ■ Lean forward and place your elbows on your knees. ■ Let your head and shoulders slump forward.
Head and shoulder drop	■ You can do the head and shoulder drop when you're sitting. ■ Let your head droop, slump your shoulders, and let your arms go limp. ■ You also can do it if you get breathless while walking. ■ Stop walking, and lean your back against a wall with your feet apart. ■ Now just slump your shoulders and relax your arms. Keep your back against the wall. Try to stay still until your breathing improves.
Supported breathing	■ Supported breathing gives your lungs more room to move and provides some comfort for you. ■ Place one or two pillows on your kitchen or dining room table. ■ Cross your arms over your chest.

(continued)

Teaching patients to decrease dyspnea
(continued)

Technique	Instructions
Supported breathing (continued)	■ Lean forward and place your arms, head, and shoulders on the pillows. Try to make your muscles loose. Stay in this position until you feel your breathing slow down.
Belly breathing	■ To perform belly breathing, let your neck and shoulders droop. ■ Rest both hands on your stomach. ■ Breathe in through your nose and let your stomach come out as far as it will. Keep your shoulders and chest relaxed. ■ Breathe out slowly through pursed lips. If you feel dizzy, take a few regular breaths before trying it again.
Imagery	■ You can make your breathing a little slower and a little easier by imagining happy times and beautiful places. ■ Find a comfortable position. Let your neck and shoulders droop. ■ Listen to your breath. ■ Close your eyes if it helps you focus. ■ Think of a favorite place that relaxes and calms you. It can be anywhere you want — watching the waves at the beach, sitting in your garden at home, or walking in a quiet forest. ■ Stay focused on that setting, keeping your body relaxed, until your breathing calms.

lows, with stuffed arms and backs, and pregnancy pillows, which support the entire body, can be perfect for dying dyspneic patients.

Repositioning also may help reduce noisy respirations. As the patient nears death and becomes unresponsive, retained oral secretions can cause the loud, gurgling respirations commonly known as a death rattle. This sound can be profoundly distressing to family members. Try repositioning the patient or raising his head with pillows; often, the noisy respirations will stop. If needed, an anticholinergic such as hyoscyamine (Levsin) or scopolamine (Scopace, Transderm Scōp) can be prescribed to help reduce the secretions.

It's even more important, however, to help families understand that their dying loved one is comfortable despite the noisy respirations and is safe from choking or suffocation. Sometimes family members ask that the patient be suctioned to remove secretions. If that happens, listen carefully to their fears, comfort them as best you can, and explain that suctioning won't eliminate the secretions and may increase the patient's distress.

Dehydration and anorexia

Stopping food and fluids is a normal part of the dying process and serves to increase the patient's comfort level. However, the process usually causes distress for family members. Explain that most dying people, especially those with end-stage cancer, rarely feel hunger or thirst. And keep these points in mind.

Dehydration in a dying person is a natural process. When this process is allowed to run its course, fluid deficits result. The need to urinate decreases. Fewer pulmonary secretions result in less coughing and choking. Fewer retained secretions means much less death rattle. Dehydration in the dying person means less edema and less pain. The vast majority of hospice nurses believe that giving intravenous fluids to dying patients is a misguided mercy that gives neither comfort nor longer life.

A similar pattern occurs with food. Less food in the stomach means less nausea and vomiting. Because a dying person's body no longer needs nutrients to fuel the activities of life, the metabolism slowly stops providing them. As a result, levels of circulating amino acids, lactic acid, and free fatty acids — compounds known to cause anorexia — increase. An altered metabolism also can make nerve cells less responsive to the decline in blood glucose level that takes place a few hours after eating, which naturally lengthens the periods between meals. Finally, changes in the level of leptin, a hormone secreted by fat cells that helps regulate weight, probably also contribute to anorexia in hospice patients.

Nausea and vomiting

The act of vomiting is controlled by the vomiting center and the chemoreceptor trigger zone (CTZ) in the brain. The CTZ contains many receptor sites for neurotransmitters such as serotonin, dopamine, and histamine, all of which may be involved in vomiting. Because the CTZ is located outside the blood-brain barrier, it can detect the presence of toxins in both the bloodstream and cerebral spinal fluid. The CTZ then sends signals to the vomiting center.

The vomiting center coordinates chemical interactions between the brain and the gastrointestinal tract. People about to vomit often look pale and feel sweaty. They may have a watery mouth from increased saliva production; they begin to retch or gag, building needed pressure to expel the stomach contents. When enough pressure has been created, the diaphragm contracts downward, the abdominal muscles tighten, the stomach becomes slack, and the esophageal sphincter opens. The final result is the rapid and forceful propulsion of stomach contents up the esophagus and out the mouth and nose. Although it's a miserable experience, once the stomach empties, the sick person typically feels better.

Besides the CTZ, the vomiting center receives information from three other pathways:
■ the cerebral cortex and limbic system, each stimulated by the senses (in particular, sight and smell) and learned associations
■ the vestibular-labyrinthine apparatus of the inner ear, which reacts to position changes
■ neurotransmitter receptors in the gut and vagus and spinal sympathetic nerves that respond to chemical stimuli in the viscera and blood.

Causes

When a patient with end-stage cancer is nauseated and vomiting, consider drug therapy and the disease itself as the most likely causes.

Adverse drug effects
Morphine and other opioids are well known for causing nausea and vomiting. When morphine is first given, it stimulates the CTZ and identifies the drug as a toxin, causing the stomach to empty. Once a steady-state level of the drug is reached, however, stimulation of the CTZ stops. Other drugs that cause nausea and vomiting include:
■ antidepressants (for depression or pain)
■ iron supplements (for fatigue and anemia)
■ NSAIDs
■ corticosteroids (for inflammation)
■ digoxin (for symptoms of heart failure).

Bowel obstruction
As tumors in the abdominal cavity grow, they compress the intestine. Tumors also may infiltrate intestinal walls. Both actions can lead to severe nausea and vomiting. Patients with end-stage ovarian, uterine, colon, or other abdominal cancers are at high risk for obstructed bowel.

Renal impairment

As many end-stage cancers progress, kidney function slowly deteriorates, leaving toxic levels in the blood, brain, and liver, prompting nausea and vomiting.

Assessment

One way to help yourself thoroughly assess the possible causes of a patient's nausea and vomiting is to assemble your questions using the mnemonic VOMIT, which stands for *vestibular; obstruction; mind; infection, inflammation, irritation; and toxins.*

To assess vestibular causes, such as motion sickness, ask questions like these: Are you dizzy? Do your ears ring? Has your hearing changed? Do you lose your balance when you get up from a chair or turn around?

To assess possible obstruction, as from constipation, ask questions like these: Is your stomach tender, painful, or bloated? When was your last bowel movement? What did it look like? Was it hard to pass? How is your appetite? Does your nausea interfere with eating? Can you drink fluids? Do you vomit after eating just a small amount of food? Do you quickly feel full? Do you have dry heaves (retching or gagging without any vomit)?

Many hospice patients feel anxious and scared. To assess causes related to the patient's mind, ask questions like these: Do you think your nausea or vomiting might be caused by your feelings? Have strong feelings ever made you feel nauseated before? What helped your nausea and vomiting in the past? Do you know of anything that causes it, such as something you eat, see, smell, breathe, or taste?

If the patient has an enlarged liver or gastroenteritis, his nausea and vomiting may result from infection, inflammation, or irritation. To find out, ask questions like these: Have you eaten something that didn't agree with you? Have you felt feverish? Do you feel sick with the flu? Does the temperature of your food or drink affect how you feel? Are cold foods or iced drinks easier to tolerate? What about hot, warm, or lukewarm?

To check for toxins as a possible cause, such as opioids or uremia, ask questions like these: Have you taken any new medications recently? Have you increased the dose of a painkiller or other medication? Are you taking your medicines more often?

Management

Like assessment, management of nausea and vomiting should follow the VOMIT mnemonic.

Vestibular causes

Antihistamines and anticholinergics can reduce nausea and vomiting stimulated by rapid head movement and other inner-ear symptoms, such as changes in hearing or ear ringing. Helping hospice patients minimize movement may help.

Obstruction

If peristalsis has stalled or the patient has squashed stomach syndrome (in which an enlarged liver or other organ presses upward against the stomach), metoclopramide (Reglan) may help. If the patient has a fecal impaction, slow, gentle, manual removal provides immediate relief.

For ongoing control of intestinal obstruction in a patient with end-stage cancer, several types of laxatives can be used, such as these:

■ a stimulant laxative, such as cascara sagrada, bisacodyl (Dulcolax), or senna (Senokot, Agoral).

■ a surfactant laxative, such as docusate (Colace, Phillip's Liqui-Gels).

■ a hyperosmolar laxative — as suppositories or mini-enemas — such as glycerin (Fleet Babylax) or lactulose

■ a saline laxative, such as magnesium hydroxide (Milk of Magnesia).

Because bulk laxatives (Metamucil, FiberCon) require extra water intake, they commonly cause feelings of fullness and shouldn't be used in patients with end-stage cancer. Neither should magnesium citrate (Citrate of Magnesia), magnesium sulfate (Epsom Salts), or mineral oil.

Mind

Anxiety-reducing drugs may be helpful, such as the benzodiazepines alprazolam (Xanax), clorazepate (Tranxene), diazepam (Valium), or lorazepam (Ativan). Environmental changes may help as well. Give the family these suggestions:

■ Avoid making meals with strong odors — such as onions, garlic, and meat.

■ Turn on kitchen fans and open windows when cooking.

■ Fresh, clean sheets and bedclothes can feel wonderful.

■ Open windows to promote cool breezes.

Infection, irritation, inflammation

Not all nausea and vomiting in patients with end-stage cancer is from progression of the disease. Sometimes these symptoms result from an irritable gastrointestinal tract. A trial of sucralfate (Carafate) or bismuth subsalicylate (Kaopectate, Pepto-Bismol) may be helpful. Nausea also may be an early sign of more serious infections, common in the dying, such as pyelonephritis, pneumonia, or central nervous system infection.

Toxins

Many drugs can cause nausea and vomiting. New-onset nausea in an end-stage cancer patient requires a drug review. If these problems are severe or continuous, an unfortunate cycle of pain and vomiting and pain may occur. Suppositories (either opioids or antiemetics) are effective in breaking this wretched cycle.

Fatigue

Almost everyone with end-stage cancer deals with substantial fatigue. It also tends to be the symptom that end-stage cancer patients find most severe and most distressing. The fatigued patient's days are spent thinking about how tired, how fatigued, and how horrible he feels.

Fatigue in end-stage cancer patients may result from electrolyte imbalances, anemia, and endocrine disturbances that occur during the dying process. As cancer progresses, metabolic processes that sustain life slowly shut down. Some drugs, once well tolerated, can cause fatigue as kidney and liver functions fail. Unresolved fear, anxiety, depression, insomnia, and poorly managed pain can also cause and worsen fatigue.

Assessment

End-stage cancer patients can rate their fatigue just like they rate pain, dyspnea, and other symptoms. Measurement tools such as the visual analog scale, numerical rating scale, and faces scale work well. Asking the patient to rate his fatigue from 0 to 10, with 0 being no fatigue and 10 being the worst fatigue imaginable, may be the easiest tool to use, since most patients have used it to rate their pain. Also ask specific questions, such as these: What makes your fatigue worse? Does a nap help? Are you less fatigued in the morning? After meals? Does activity make it worse? Does anything help?

Management

Various drugs can be used to manage fatigue in patients with end-stage cancer, including corticosteroids, psychostimulants, and antidepressants. (See *How drugs reduce fatigue.*) Dexamethasone (Decadron) is the corticosteroid used most often. Psychostimulants include methylphenidate (Ritalin), dextroamphetamine (Dexedrine), pemoline (Cylert), and modafinil (Provigil).

Antidepressant therapy may employ a selective serotonin reuptake inhibitor or a tricyclic antidepressant. The former most often involves citalopram (Celexa), paroxetine (Paxil), fluoxetine (Prozac), or sertraline (Zoloft). The latter most often involves amitriptyline (Elavil) or desipramine (Norpramin). However, these drugs may take 4 to 5 weeks to reach therapeutic levels and effects.

How drugs reduce fatigue

Drug type	Drug effects
Corticosteroids	▪ Increase feelings of well-being ▪ Increase energy levels
Psychostimulants	▪ Typically increase energy and well-being ▪ Improve cognition and concentration ▪ Modafinil (Provigil) may reduce fatigue in multiple sclerosis
Selective serotonin reuptake inhibitors	▪ May elevate mood and provide energizing effects
Tricyclic antidepressants	▪ May elevate mood and relieve neuropathic pain

Sleep problems

Poor sleep often accompanies fatigue in end-stage cancer patients. Many fear falling asleep and never waking up. On days where the end-stage cancer seems to be taking control (pain escalates, nausea increases, or bowels become impacted), it may take great courage to fall asleep. Many hospice patients report having complex, vivid, highly detailed dreams. They may have nightmares or night terrors. They may dream of people they need or want to contact. They may dream of friends and family members who have already died.

Several drugs may help combat sleep problems. Some of these sleep aids are benzodiazepines; others aren't. (See *Comparing sleep aids*, page 122.) Remember that benzodiazepines may increase existing depression; they also may increase constipation and cause dry mouth, lethargy, apathy, and fatigue. Adverse effects of the nonbenzodiazepine sleep aids, although rare, may include nausea, dizziness, nightmares, headache, irritability, and vision changes.

Certain herbal supplements may improve sleep, particularly melatonin, valerian, hops, and wild lettuce. The best results may come from taking valerian and hops together or taking melatonin. Melatonin products labeled "natural, bovine, or organic" may contain viruses or non-medical ingredi-

Comparing sleep aids

Drug	Half-life	Onset of sleep
Benzodiazepines		
estazolam (ProSom)	8–24 hours	45–60 minutes
temazepam (Restoril)	8–20 hours	Varies
triazolam (Halcion)	2–6 hours	Varies
Nonbenzodiazepines		
zaleplon (Sonata)	1 hour	45–60 minutes
zolpidem (Ambien)	2.6 hours	15–45 minutes

ents. Only synthetic melatonin should be used. Keep in mind that valerian has a foul odor (like smelly feet) and can cause vivid dreams. Also, make sure the patient takes standardized herbs from a reputable company.

Other nondrug treatments may improve sleep as well, including these.

■ Giving supplemental oxygen at 2 L/minute by nasal cannula at night may improve sleep by reducing anxiety.

■ A warm tub bath or bed bath promotes relaxation.

■ Washing the patient's hands and face with warm soapy water at bedtime can feel soothing and relaxing.

■ Try gentle back rubs or hand massages with warmed lotion.

■ A cup of warm milk helps promote sleep. So does hot decaffeinated tea and plain hot water with a slice of lemon.

■ Make the day stimulating to help the patient be ready for resting at night. For instance, as appropriate, encourage the patient to visit with friends, talk on the telephone, dictate letters, take short day trips, sit outside, play with pets, look at works of art in a museum or a book, and play board games or card games.

■ Set up a sleep and wake schedule, and decide on a bedtime and times for daytime naps as well as a consistent awakening time.

■ Play quiet, soothing music to relax the patient before bed.

■ If the patient is afraid to go to sleep, prayer or meditation can help dramatically. Or try reading from a spiritual book of the patient's choosing.

Managing emergencies

As a patient with cancer nears the end of his life, several emergent conditions may arise. They include hypercalcemia of malignancy, pathologic fractures, spinal cord compression, bleeding, skin lesions, seizures, terminal restlessness, suffering, and nearing-death awareness.

Hypercalcemia of malignancy

Normally, almost all of the body's calcium stores are banked in bone. As metastases destroy bone, calcium is released into the bloodstream. Symptoms include excessive thirst, muscle weakness, nausea, vomiting, loss of appetite, lethargy, fatigue, and confusion. Hydration dilutes the serum calcium level and increases urinary output of calcium. Mobility is also helpful in promoting resorption of serum calcium. For mild-to-moderate elevations of calcium, patients should try to increase their oral intake of fluids to 3 to 4 liters of water per day and maintain their mobility.

Severe hypercalcemia can be treated in different ways. A patient severely compromised by his disease and nearing end of life may not want to be treated. In this case, symptomatic care with laxatives, antiemetics, and antipsychotics or anxiolytics for mental changes may be sufficient. A patient who is still active and can expect a significant number of weeks or months of good quality of life may choose active treatment. Immediately begin hydrating the patient with intravenous saline solution, preferably in an inpatient setting. Loop diuretics such as furosemide (Lasix) cause the kidneys to excrete more calcium. Increasing fluid intake and the use of loop diuretics can bring down corrected total serum calcium levels in the short run, however, the bisphosphonates are newer treatments. Pamidronate disodium (Aredia), an I.V. drug, is the first choice for long-term calcium reduction to lessen symptoms and improve quality of life.

Pathologic fractures

In end-stage cancer patients, pathologic fractures occur when bony metastases invade bones near joints. The most common site is the weight-bearing femoral neck. Treatment depends, as always, on the individual patient. Goals include pain relief and restored mobility. Surgical repair (most often with pins or a rod) offers the quickest pain management, even in patients unable to ambulate. However, conservative treatment (skin traction, regional blocks, use of pillows for positioning) can be equally effective for some patients, depending on the fracture location and the patient's overall health status.

Spinal cord compression

Spinal cord compression occurs in 5% to 30% of cancer patients. It's most common in patients with advanced disease and is most likely in patients with lung, breast, or prostate cancers. It happens most often when a metastatic tumor growing on the bony structure of the vertebrae infiltrates the epidural space and presses on the dura, the tough membrane that covers the spinal cord. As the tumor grows, the resulting symptoms depend on where the tumor presses on the spinal cord and how much the cord is compressed. Symptoms include leg weakness, loss of bowel and bladder control, sensory changes (feeling pins and needles, numbness, and hypersensitivity of the skin), positive Babinski's reflex, sexual dysfunction, and paralysis.

Treatment options include corticosteroids, radiation therapy, and surgery. The most common hospice treatment is dexamethasone (Decadron), which decreases swelling in the spinal cord, reduces pain, and helps preserve neurologic function.

Bleeding

Bleeding may result from tumor invasion, systemic processes such as disseminated intravascular coagulopathy, or abnormalities in platelet functioning. Hemorrhaging can occur as hematemesis, melena, hemoptysis, hematuria, epistaxis, vaginal bleeding, or ulcerated skin lesions. The hemorrhage may be an acute catastrophic event, episodic major bleeds, or ongoing low-volume oozing. In patients with end-stage cancer, treatment that stops the bleeding without providing full resuscitative measures is most appropriate.

When an end-stage cancer patient is at risk for a major hemorrhage, family members and caregivers need to be sensitively informed and prepared because these events can be extremely distressing. Using dark towels to absorb blood, applying pressure to the site of hemorrhaging, and placing patients in the lateral position are simple empowering measures. A rapid-acting sedative should be available for sedation, such as midazolam 2.5 mg given subcutaneously.

Skin lesions

The wounds of terminally ill patients won't heal or improve. Care should focus on palliation and keeping the patient comfortable, clean, and odor free. This may involve treating pain, bleeding, oozing, necrosis, or infection at the wound or tumor site. Existing wounds may worsen or new wounds may develop, partly because the patient is eating less. As a result, the patient's serum albumin levels fall and rapid skin breakdown occurs, especially on bony prominences and areas of unrelieved pressure. The problem is worsened because dying patients move less often and are unable to reposition themselves to lessen pressure during sleep.

Wounds themselves may be a sign of impending death. The skin is an organ, and when it's not properly perfused, it dies. A patient who had no skin breakdown may suddenly develop a large black ulcer, most often on the sacrum. Patients usually die within 14 days of the appearance of a terminal ulcer, sometimes within 24 hours.

Old viral infections can be re-activated with lowered immune function and appear as painful shingles, genital herpes, or other viral infections. Caregivers should double glove when caring for patients with open lesions, vesicles, or infections.

Cancer-related wounds

Many types of wounds result from cancer. Wounds may be related to surgery, radiation treatment, or complications of cancer progression, such as fistulas, externalized tumors, or other metastasis. Cancer can spread to adjacent tissue or travel to other sites via blood or lymph vessels. Surgical sites, whether from a cancer resection or from an unrelated procedure, are prime targets for metastases because of increased blood flow and growth factors for healing in the area at the site of the cancer. In patients with cancer in remission, incisions from unrelated surgeries may develop metastases from a distant primary tumor. Abdominal cancers can spread along ligaments in the torso and emerge at the umbilicus. This form of metastasis can cause problems even before the tumor externalizes. The patient often has onset of bleeding from the umbilicus.

Fistulas Providing wound care to oncology patients is challenging because the size and shape of the wounds change and fistulas may develop. Draining fistulas should be pouched whenever possible to collect the drainage, avoid damage to healthy adjacent tissue, and prevent odor. The drainage can be caustic if the fistula acts as an ileostomy. If there's copious drainage, it should be directed away from the patient by using an ileostomy pouch and connector tube, which allows the drainage to be diverted to a urine collection bag. Fistulas may not be easily pouched like an ostomy site; they're irregular and change size and shape frequently, or may be recessed.

Tumors Tumors exposed to air also create problems. Tumors bleed, drain, stick to bandages, cause odor, and are difficult to dress. Removing bandaging can be painful if tumor tissue is disturbed in the process. To minimize problems, protect the tumor with a hydrophilic cream and then cover it with a layer of Vaseline gauze and cover that with an absorbent dressing. Or use an alginate dressing that's easily rinsed off and has hemostatic and anti-infective properties. If there's copious drainage or bleeding, the dressing can be held in place with Montgomery straps to avoid tape burns and trauma to the surrounding skin from frequent dressing changes. For an ambulatory patient who doesn't want his clothing soiled, a disposable diaper or incontinence pad can be used as a dressing topper to provide a waterproof layer.

These tumors are also prone to anaerobic or fungal infections, which are usually superficial but can be deep. Odor is often the first sign of an anaerobic infection. Superficial infections can be treated with metronidazole (MetroCream) or silver sulfadiazine (Silvadene). Deep infections require systemic metronidazole. When a wound isn't healing, povidone may be used to keep the wound clean, but this can be painful for some patients.

Skin around the mouth or perineal area may develop candidiasis (thrush) particularly in patients with reduced immunity as a result of chemotherapy, drug- or illness-induced dry mouth, or diabetes. Thrush of the oropharynx or esophagus may also occur in these patients. Treat external lesions with nystatin (Mycostatin) or clotrimazole (Lotrimin). Mild oropharyngeal and esophageal lesions can be treated with either a nystatin suspension using a "swish and swallow" technique, or clotrimazole troches. Patients with low fluid intake typically don't tolerate the troches. Systemic therapy can be used for more severe cases when the patient is in a lot of pain; drugs include fluconazole (Diflucan) and itraconazole (Sporanox).

External tumor that has been destroyed by radiation may "dry up" and die. Dead pieces of the tumor may painlessly break away. The best way to treat skin damaged by radiation hasn't been determined. Use caution if you apply petrolatum-like products to these wounds.

Seizures

Primary or metastatic brain tumors may cause seizures. Electrolyte imbalances and metabolic changes as end-stage cancer progresses also may contribute to seizures. To control them, give diazepam (Valium) by rectum, either by suppository or oral tablet placed against the rectal mucosa. This treatment may begin if the seizures are new and the patient is nearing death. Some patients may already be receiving oral phenytoin (Dilantin), which can be continued by suppository when the patient is unable to swallow.

Also, teach family members how to keep the patient safe during a seizure. Status epilepticus, a continuous seizure accompanied by respiratory distress, is an emergency. Plans for how to handle this problem should be made according to the patient's prognosis and performance status.

Terminal restlessness

Sometimes referred to as terminal agitation, terminal anguish, terminal delirium, or hyper-alertness, this emergency most often starts as agitation that rapidly increases. Other symptoms follow, including purposeful motor activity, muscle twitching, spasticity, fitful sleep and rest patterns, and escalating anxiety. This condition most often comes on quickly, occurring as the patient is actively dying.

Causes are numerous and include rapidly escalating pain, kidney failure, liver failure, electrolyte imbalances, polypharmacy, sensory overload, urine retention, fecal impaction, hypoxia, emotional distress (suffering, fear, unfinished business, guilt, regret), inability to communicate, and alcohol withdrawal. Interventions include elimination of the cause if possible (such as oxygen for hypoxia or removal of fecal impaction). The patient may need combination drug therapy to control this emergency, including a sedative such as midazolam (Versed), phenobarbital (Solfoton), or pentobarbital (Nembutal).

Suffering

Even if the physical symptoms of dying are managed well, emotional, spiritual, and psychosocial symptoms can be overwhelming to both end-stage cancer patients and those who love and care for them. End-of-life research has shown that dying patients who feel their lives have had no meaning are at higher risk of suffering. The alienation and isolation of dying and poorly managed pain and other symptoms add to suffering.

While the temptation may be strong among hospice nurses to devalue the suffering of end-stage cancer patients and their families simply because there seems little we can do, this might add to the patient's anguish. A willingness to connect and establish a trusting relationship with the patient and family is an effective way to help ease suffering. Simply bearing witness to someone's suffering has been shown to reduce it.

Bearing witness to suffering does not mean that you need to engage in inappropriate interactions, camping out at a dying patient's home 24 hours a day or holding the hand of a distraught spouse or child. Involvement in an end-stage cancer patient's suffering requires a high degree of professionalism and a willingness to accept the patient and family where they are. The power of presence can't be overstated.

Nearing-death awareness

A special knowledge and sometimes control over the process of dying is fairly common in the final weeks, days, and hours of life. It is especially common in patients dying of end-stage cancer. Nearing-death awareness is most often not a true problem or symptom for the patient. For families, however, witnessing their dying loved one converse with long-deceased Uncle Harry can be very frightening.

Nearing-death awareness is much different than near-death experiences. Those who have had a near-death experience typically do so as a result of an acute physical trauma, such as electrocution, cardiac arrest, or a serious motor vehicle accident. These patients were at the brink of death and then brought back. Their accounts are often very similar and often include out-of-body sensations, bright lights at the end of a dark tunnel, the presence of dead loved ones, and the appearance of God, Jesus, and angels. Most often, near-death experiences have lasting, profound emotional and spiritual effects.

In contrast, nearing-death awareness is not an acute experience. It's gradual. The dying patient may tell caregivers that it's time to call friends and family, that the end is near. Vivid and symbolic dreams may relay ways to complete unfinished business, reduce anxieties, and calm fears. The patient may describe a place not visible to others. He may communicate seemingly illogical messages or speak to nonexistent people. Travel and a change in scenery is often mentioned. Dying patients may feel a need to find maps, pack suitcases, or buy airplane tickets. Getting in lines and standing at a gate or a door are frequent scenarios in dying patients who are experiencing nearing-death awareness. This may go on for several days.

If a dying patient has specific needs, such as reconciliation with an estranged friend or family member, these needs may be expressed clearly or metaphorically. Choosing a time that is "right" is another manifestation of nearing-death awareness. Some dying patients wait to die until certain people arrive or leave the room, or until they feel certain those they are leaving behind will eventually be alright.

It's tempting to chalk these episodes up to confusion or too much morphine. However, research is continuing to suggest that nearing-death awareness is a complex and important aspect of dying not connected to cognition or drug therapy.

Patients with heart failure | 9

About 5 million Americans have heart failure and, despite advances in treatment, deaths from heart failure continue to rise. About 1 in 4 people die within 1 year of being diagnosed, many from sudden cardiac death. The rest decline more slowly, with symptoms increasing as cardiac function decreases.

Palliative care—managing the symptoms and enhancing quality of life rather than attempting to cure the disease—is a critical focus of the care that heart failure patients should receive. However, because remissions and exacerbations are common in this disorder, it can be difficult to predict an appropriate time for end-of-life care to begin. Consequently, palliative care should be in your mind whenever you care for a patient with heart failure.

To start, make sure you understand key facts about what happens in heart failure and how the disorder progresses. Then, be ready to discuss the patient's treatment goals, relieve symptoms as much as possible, address any concurrent illnesses, attend to the patient's psychosocial and spiritual needs, and discuss his end-of-life goals.

Understanding heart failure

Heart failure is a complex condition that results from any structural or functional heart disease that reduces ejection fraction—the percentage of blood in the heart that's expelled with each ventricular contraction. Usually, heart failure results from impaired function of the left ventricle. It also may result from diseases of the pericardium, myocardium, endocardium, or great vessels. Coronary artery disease, hypertension, valvular heart disease, and dilated cardiomyopathy are common causes of heart failure.

No matter what the cause of heart failure, if ejection fraction declines too far, the body's need for oxygen goes unmet and the patient develops dyspnea, fatigue, and other symptoms. (See *Symptoms of heart failure*, page

Symptoms of heart failure

Type of heart failure	Symptoms
Left-sided	Cough Frothy, pink expectorant Nocturnal dyspnea (orthopnea) Rales (alveolar edema) Shortness of breath, tachypnea
Right-sided	Ascites Generalized venous engorgement Hepatomegaly Jugular vein distension Peripheral edema Serous effusions in body cavities
Both	Exertional dyspnea Gallop rhythm Poor peripheral perfusion Tachycardia Weakness and fatigue Weight loss

130.) Keep in mind, however, that symptoms may not always match the degree of ventricular impairment. Some patients have symptoms of heart failure with a normal-size left ventricle and normal ejection fraction (diastolic dysfunction); others have symptoms only with severe left ventricular dilation, markedly reduced ejection fraction, or both (systolic dysfunction).

The New York Heart Association (NYHA) classification provides a system for categorizing heart failure patients functionally and therapeutically. (See *New York Heart Association classification of heart failure*.) It's the most widely used scale, although it's relatively insensitive to important changes in activity tolerance. The six-minute walk test, measurement of the distance a patient can walk in six minutes, may have more prognostic significance and may help in assessing functional capacity in end-stage heart failure.

Determining end-stage heart failure

Management of heart failure at all stages involves a substantial palliative component. However, determining the appropriate time to start end-of-life care can be quite difficult. Age may affect the patient's treatment goals because younger patients may be better candidates for heart transplantation; older patients are more likely to be referred for hospice care.

New York Heart Association classification of heart failure

Class	Characteristics
I	■ No limitation of activities ■ No symptoms with ordinary activities
II	■ Slight, mild limitation of activity ■ Comfortable at rest or with mild exertion
III	■ Marked limitation of activity ■ Comfortable only at rest
IV	■ Discomfort and symptoms with any activity ■ Should be at complete rest, confined to bed or chair

 LIFESPAN Suffering caused by heart failure is more substantial among elderly patients, placing them at greater risk for poorer outcomes. Elderly patients experience psychological distress, decreased cognitive and social function, and recurring symptoms that reduce their quality of life.

There are no set criteria for determining when a patient has advanced to the end stages of heart failure. A patient with refractory heart failure may be referred to a clinic that specializes in heart failure treatment to make sure that medical management is optimized and that all viable surgical options have been considered.

As a general rule of thumb, patients may need a referral to palliative care if they have NYHA Class IV heart failure, an ejection fraction less than 25% despite optimal treatment, a 6-minute walk distance of less than 300 meters, symptoms that interfere with activities of daily living, and several of these prognostic indicators:

■ decreasing left ventricular ejection fraction, peak exercise oxygen uptake, and hematocrit
■ worsening NYHA functional status
■ severe hyponatremia
■ widening QRS on a 12-lead electrocardiogram
■ chronic hypotension
■ resting tachycardia
■ renal insufficiency
■ intolerance of conventional therapy
■ refractory volume overload.

Stages of heart failure

Stage	Myocardial structure changes	Patient's conditions
A		
High risk for heart failure	No	Atherosclerosis Diabetes mellitus Hypertension Metabolic syndrome Obesity
B		
Asymptomatic heart failure	Yes	Previous myocardial infarction Left ventricular dysfunction Valvular disease
C		
Symptomatic heart failure	Yes	Above plus symptoms of heart failure
D		
Refractory end-stage heart failure	Yes	Refractory heart failure requiring specialized interventions

Two or three hospital admissions for heart failure in the previous year support a need for referral along with the patient fitting stage D heart failure on the scale developed by the American Heart Association and the American College of Cardiologists. (See *Stages of heart failure.*) This scale includes changes in ventricular structure, which is a hallmark of heart failure. The ventricular chamber dilates or hypertrophies and becomes more spherical in a process called cardiac remodeling. Usually, remodeling precedes the development of symptoms.

To help your heart failure patient receive the care he needs, assess his condition carefully, and provide comprehensive palliative care according to the patient's symptoms and individual challenges. The goals of palliative care include the relief of suffering, management and control of symptoms, and improvement of functional capacity and quality of life.

Symptoms	Treatment
None	■ Risk reduction ■ ACE inhibitor or angiotensin receptor blocker, as needed
Symptoms with mild exertion	■ Stage A treatments ■ Beta blocker, as needed
Shortness of breath, fatigue, reduced exercise tolerance	■ Stage A and B treatments ■ Diuretic ■ Dietary sodium restriction
Marked symptoms at rest despite maximum medical therapy	■ Stage A, B, and C treatments ■ Consideration of palliative or hospice care

LIFESPAN Heart failure may develop in a child as a result of a congenital heart defect or an acquired heart problem such as rheumatic valve disease. If surgical and drug treatments fail, parents must make excruciating decisions about whether to continue aggressive treatment or adopt a more palliative approach. A team of professionals can help the parents and child cope with the chronic illness and crises of life with a severe cardiac disorder. In addition to physicians and nurses, the team may include a psychologist, chaplain, social worker, recreational therapist, art therapist, music therapist, physical therapist, and others to help ensure comfort and quality of life.

Assessment

Two of the most important areas to assess in a patient with heart failure are functional capacity and volume status.

Functional capacity

To assess functional capacity, look at the type, severity, and duration of symptoms that occur during activities of daily living and that may impair the patient's ability to pursue them. Ask your patient whether he can perform routine tasks, such as dressing, bathing, climbing stairs, and doing chores, without stopping. Ask whether there are activities he used to perform but no longer can. Changes in the patient's ability to perform daily activities typically relate closely to important changes in clinical status.

Volume status

Your assessment of volume status is critically important because, among other things, it determines the need for changes to the patient's diet and drug regimen. At each physical exam, assess and record the patient's body weight, sitting and standing blood pressures, jugular vein distension, severity of organ congestion, and amount of peripheral edema.

The most reliable sign of volume overload is jugular vein distension. A positive hepatojugular reflux indicates elevated filling pressures. Most patients with peripheral edema should be considered fluid overloaded; however, noncardiac causes need to be considered and evaluated.

Although body weight may be the best indicator of fluid status in the early stages of heart failure, it's a less reliable indicator in the later stages. End-stage heart failure patients may accumulate non-fluid weight or may lose muscle mass and body fat from cardiac cachexia. Also, patients with end-stage heart failure and volume overload may show signs of hypoperfusion, rare at earlier stages. These include:

- narrowed pulse pressure
- cool extremities
- altered mentation
- Cheyne-Stokes respirations
- resting tachycardia
- increased ratio of blood urea nitrogen to creatinine.

Treatment

When your assessment has confirmed the advancement of the patient's heart failure, you'll need to sit down with the patient and family to discuss their expectations and the goals of care. This discussion should cover a wide range of topics, such as symptom management outcomes, treatment options, and the desire for palliative and hospice care.

Talk about expected treatment outcomes, the burden of treatment, and the impact of treatment on the patient's quality of life. Ask the patient where he'd like to receive care and what kinds of treatments he desires. Talk about the poor outcomes for cardiopulmonary resuscitation in patients with end-stage heart failure—a topic that can lead naturally to discussion of advance directives. Patients with the most severe symptoms commonly prefer to trade time for symptom relief. Finally, reassure the patient and family that you'll provide frequent updates on prognosis, care goals, and treatment planning.

The goals of treatment are to reduce cardiac workload while improving oxygen delivery and pump function. Many components may be included in the plan to reach this goal. (See *Treating heart failure*.) Carefully tailored drug therapy is one of the most important.

Drug therapy

Several drug types can be used to treat heart failure based on the patient's individual needs. (See *Drugs for heart failure*, page 136.) In end-stage heart failure, it's important to make sure that patients are at the target level of these drugs or at the largest dose tolerated in keeping with the patient's wishes.

Treating heart failure

Patients, family members, and the care team can use several measures to maximize function, comfort, and quality of life in patients with heart failure.

- Complying with drug therapy
- Avoiding sodium and excess fluids
- Adhering to low-fat, low-cholesterol diet
- Managing symptoms
- Checking weight regularly
- Exercising as tolerated
- Managing anxiety and depression
- Providing teaching
- Attending to spiritual needs

Drugs for heart failure

Drug	Effects
Angiotensin converting enzyme (ACE) inhibitors	■ Prevent angiotensin II increase. ■ Prevent cardiac remodeling. ■ Reduce preload and afterload.
Angiotensin receptor blockers	■ Prevent angiotensin II increase through different pathway than ACE inhibitors. ■ Similar neurohormonal effects as ACE inhibitors.
Beta blockers	■ Reduce effects of sympathetic nervous system on heart (increased myocardial oxygen demand, increased preload and afterload). ■ Reverse cardiac remodeling.
Aldosterone antagonists	■ Block sodium retention. ■ Block cardiac remodeling.
Diuretics	■ Reduce volume overload. ■ Reduce pulmonary and peripheral edema.
Digitalis	■ Provides neurohormonal modulation.
Nitrates	■ May be indicated for patients who can't tolerate ACE inhibitors or angiotensin receptor blockers because of impaired renal function or patients already receiving maximum therapy to improve cardiac output, volume overload, or cardiac remodeling.

If the patient has persistent severe hypotension, eliminate as many drugs known to cause it as possible without compromising the patient's functional capacity and cardiac health. Consider reducing the angiotensin-converting enzyme inhibitor, angiotensin receptor blocker, and beta blocker. Avoid or, if needed, withdraw drugs known to adversely affect patients with heart failure, including:

■ nonsteroidal anti-inflammatory drugs
■ most antiarrhythmics
■ most calcium channel blockers
■ hormone therapies other than those used to treat hormone deficiencies
■ some herbal supplements
■ nutritional supplements used to treat heart failure.

Meticulous fluid management is critical in end-stage heart failure. If the patient develops resistance to diuretic therapy, you may need to give an increased or divided intravenous dose of the prescribed diuretic. Or the patient may benefit from switching to a loop diuretic to improve drug availability or adding a thaizide diuretic to the regimen. In addition, the patient should follow a sodium-restricted diet. Weigh the patient daily to check for fluid retention, and assess and manage the likely causes of retained fluid.

Use opioids, anxiolytics, and sleep aids to ease pain and distress and provide compassionate care. (See *Not just a pain reliever*, page 138.) Don't preclude the use of intravenous inotropes and diuretics for palliation in end-stage patients, although long-term use of an intravenous inotropic is indicated only for patients who can't be stabilized with other optimal medical therapy.

Other interventions

Additional interventions that may improve heart failure symptoms include exercise training and cardiac resynchronization therapy. Exercise training is beneficial in ambulatory patients, improving both physical and psychological status. Cardiac resynchronization therapy is beneficial for patients with an ejection fraction of 35% or less, no sinus rhythm, Class III or IV heart failure, and a prolonged QRS interval despite optimal medical therapy.

Also, carefully assess and treat disorders that may aggravate the patient's heart failure. For example, addressing issues such as sleep-disordered breathing and anemia can help patients feel more rested, less fatigued, and generally improved. Use of continuous or bilevel positive airway pressure (commonly known as CPAP or BiPAP) may improve nighttime sleep and reduce daytime sleepiness, a common complaint.

Psychological care

Advanced heart failure affects the quality of a patient's entire life, including its physical, emotional, social, spiritual, and cognitive aspects. Physical ability, role performance, mental function, social interactions, and general health perceptions are all increasingly challenged as the patient's illness advances. It's no wonder, then, that heart failure commonly causes substantial psychological distress and may lead to depression and anxiety.

Depression

In fact, we know that patients with heart failure have higher rates of depression than the general population. Between 11% and 25% of outpatients with heart failure develop depression; between 35% and 70% of inpatients develop it. Most depressed heart failure patients receive no treatment for their depression, and they're no more likely to see a mental health specialist than patients who aren't depressed. Depression and anxiety tend to increase and peak between 1 month and 3 days before death.

EXPERT INSIGHTS

Not just a pain reliever

I'm caring for a nursing home resident with end-stage heart failure and pulmonary edema. He's tachypneic at 32 breaths/minute and has a look of terror in his eyes. I called the attending physician and requested small, frequent doses of oral morphine. She refused, saying, "He's not in pain, so morphine isn't indicated."

I believe a small dose of morphine would make this patient more comfortable and less panicky. Am I wrong? — D.P., Tenn.

No. It's the physician who needs a refresher course in Pharmacology 101. Morphine does much more than simply relieve pain. Because it acts as a vasodilator, it can increase cardiac output. It's also a respiratory depressant, so it suppresses the horrible drowning sensation your patient is experiencing while decreasing the respiratory drive for that next, precious breath. When oral morphine is provided for patients like yours, arterial blood gas values actually improve, proving the efficacy of morphine for dyspnea. Finally, morphine can produce a mild, but welcome, euphoria, relieving feelings of terror and panic.

I applaud you for your commitment to patient advocacy. Contact the physician again and request 5 mg of liquid morphine every 4 hours, as needed. If she still balks, go through channels to the medical director, if necessary, to get your patient the treatment he needs to relieve his suffering.

— JOY UFEMA, RN, MS

We also know that depression affects prognosis in patients with heart failure and is an important outcome in evaluating heart failure therapy. The diagnosis of depression has an independent link with mortality, quality of life, and functional status. Clearly, treating a heart failure patient's depression holds promise for improving his quality of life.

Depression is measured clinically using one of two methods: symptom count instruments and depression assessment scales. The symptom count instruments classify depression by counting the number of depressive symptoms the person displays. (See *Counting symptoms of depression.*) You also can assess your patient for depression using a standardized depression assessment scale.

The two main modes of treatment for depression are drug therapy and psychotherapy. Patient education, exercise, social support, and family care also can reduce symptoms of depression. Referral to a mental health

Counting symptoms of depression

One way to assess your patient's depression is by counting his symptoms and applying the result to the scoring system described here.

Symptoms
- Depressed mood most of the day nearly every day
- Markedly reduced interest and pleasure in most activities, most days
- Significant weight loss or gain
- Insomnia or hypersomnia
- Psychomotor agitation and retardation
- Impaired concentration, indecisiveness
- Recurrent thoughts of death or suicide
- Feelings of worthlessness or guilt
- Fatigue, loss of energy

Scores
If your patient has five of these symptoms nearly every day for 2 weeks or more, he most likely has major depression. If he has two to four of these symptoms nearly every day for 2 weeks , he probably has minor depression. If he has three or four of these symptoms for a protracted time — more than 2 years — he probably has a type of chronic depression known as dysthymia.

provider for psychotherapy may be enough to help the patient develop the coping skills he needs not only for his heart failure but for his impending death.

Some patients benefit from drug therapy, particularly those with:
- severe depression
- chronic or recurrent depression
- depression with psychotic features
- a history of positive response to drug therapy
- a family history of depression
- inability to pursue psychotherapy.

For a patient who needs drug therapy, treatment usually is with a selective serotonin reuptake inhibitor (SSRI) or tricyclic antidepressant. SSRIs seem to have no effect on blood pressure or arrhythmias and little effect on conduction and ECG intervals. Tricyclic antidepressants cause more adverse effects, are contraindicated in patients with ischemic disease, and should be used cautiously in all patients with a history of significant heart disease.

Anxiety

Anxiety is a normal reaction to stress; however, it may become an excessive, irrational dread of everyday situations manifesting as a state of fear, apprehension, dread, and foreboding. Anxiety affects up to two-thirds of patients with heart failure. Signs and symptoms of anxiety may include anorexia, chest pain, palpitations, tachycardia, nausea, vomiting, diarrhea, urinary frequency, dizziness, faintness, dry mouth, dyspnea, hyperventilation, and flushing. Treatment may include drug therapy, biofeedback, and psychotherapy.

Spiritual care

Spirituality is an experiential process that involves a quest for meaning and purpose, transcendence (a sense that being human is more than material existence), connectedness (with others, with nature, with divinity) and values (such as justice). Spirituality influences adaptation to illness.

In patients with heart failure, hope is positively related to social function; patients who are more hopeful maintain involvement in life regardless of the physical limitations imposed by the disease. In studies, patients described a three-step process in which spirituality eased their adjustment to heart failure:

■ development of regret about past behaviors and lifestyles
■ search for meaning in the present experience of heart failure
■ search for hope for the future and the reclaiming of optimism.

In a group of heart failure patients awaiting transplantation, faith in God was one of the top 10 areas of life with which they were most satisfied. But whether or not patients and caregivers hold religious beliefs, they almost all express needs for love, meaning, purpose, and sometimes transcendence.

You can assess your patient's sense of spirituality and need to pursue spirituality using one of several standardized questionnaires. Important interventions include obtaining a spiritual history; being with the patient and family; listening to the patient's fears, hopes, pain, and dreams; paying attention to body, mind, and spirit integration; incorporating the patient's spiritual or religious practices, as appropriate; and soliciting the services of clergy or another spiritual advisor of the patient's choosing.

Spiritual coping may be displayed by the patient's hope for finishing important goals and a peaceful death, a sense of control, acceptance of and strength to deal with the situation, and a sense of meaning and purpose to life in the midst of suffering.

Patients in end-stage heart failure need your support for daily living and psychological and spiritual issues and your assurance of continuity of care across care settings. Patients and families also need your help in making difficult medical decisions and making sure their wishes for care are followed. With attentive care, you can accomplish these goals and make sure that the patient's suffering is relieved, his symptoms managed, and his functional capacity and quality of life improved.

Patients with neurologic disease

10

Several neurologic disorders follow a degenerative course that eventually results in the patient's death. These disorders impact quality of life for both patients and families, in some cases for decades. These disorders present a challenge to health care providers seeking to both manage the symptoms and determine an appropriate time to refer the patient to a palliative care team and, later, to a hospice program. Although determining a realistic six-month prognosis is difficult, it's possible to ease the patient's symptoms and support the patient's family as these diseases reach their final stages.

This chapter reviews three terminal neurologic disorders: amyotrophic lateral sclerosis (ALS), Alzheimer's disease, and Huntington's disease.

Amyotrophic lateral sclerosis

ALS is a progressive, degenerative disease. It's also known as Lou Gehrig's disease, after the popular New York Yankee baseball player who was diagnosed with it. ALS is the most common motor neuron disease in the United States, with about 5,000 new cases diagnosed each year. It's more common in men and usually is diagnosed between ages 40 and 60. About half of those who develop ALS die within 2 to 5 years after symptoms start, usually from respiratory failure. (See *Theories about amyotrophic lateral sclerosis*, page 142.)

Progressive symptoms

Symptoms of ALS result from the degeneration and demyelination of motor neurons in the anterior horn of the spinal cord, brain stem, and cerebral cor-

Theories about amyotrophic lateral sclerosis

We don't know a great deal about what causes amyotrophic lateral sclerosis (ALS) or what makes it progress. Here are some theories.

The disease may have a genetic component. Familial ALS, linked to chromosome 21 defects, makes up about 5% to 10% of cases. The rest are known as the sporadic form and include no family history.

ALS also may have metabolic or viral roots. Abnormal glutamate metabolism and hydrogen peroxide production may be involved. And echovirus RNA has been isolated in spinal cord tissue in some people with the nonfamilial form.

ALS also has been linked to oxidative stress and cellular damage — as have Alzheimer's disease and Parkinson's disease. Neurons are easily damaged by oxygen-free radicals and the activation of immune cells that propagate further cellular injury.

Other variables include environmental influences, excess intracellular calcium, and antibodies to calcium channels.

tex. Upper motor neuron dysfunction causes spastic, weak muscles with fasciculations and increased deep tendon reflexes. Lower motor neuron dysfunction causes muscle flaccidity, paresis, paralysis, and atrophy. Death of the motor neurons results in axonal degeneration, demyelination, glial proliferation, and scarring along the corticospinal tract.

Initially, ALS causes weakness and paresis that may affect only one muscle group. Early in the disease, surviving motor neurons sprout new branches to affected muscle fibers, which preserves muscle strength. However, when more than half of lower motor neurons are affected, this process fails, and weakness becomes detectable. It typically affects the hands first, then the upper arms and shoulders, and finally the legs. Continued brainstem involvement leads to progressive atrophy of the tongue and facial muscles and eventually to dysphagia and dysarthria. As the frontal lobe becomes involved, emotional lability and loss of control may result, but vision, hearing, sensation, and cognitive ability usually remain intact.

Diagnosis and treatment

ALS is a diagnosis of exclusion based on the patient's signs and symptoms. Electromyography, nerve conduction studies, magnetic resonance imaging, and blood testing may be used to rule out other disorders, such as multiple sclerosis, brain and spinal cord tumors, infection by human immunodeficiency virus, and Lyme disease.

Riluzole (Rilutek), a glutamate inhibitor, is the only drug currently used for ALS. It doesn't cure the disease but may prolong life for several months and delay the need for mechanical ventilation.

Patients with ALS benefit from multidisciplinary care that seeks to prevent the complications of immobility and to address the physical and psychological needs of patient and family.

Alzheimer's disease

Alzheimer's disease is a form of dementia marked by progressive deterioration of intellectual function, emotional control, social behavior, and motivation. The progression rate varies, but eventually the patient will be unable to make judgments and care for himself. Patients may live many years with the disorder, but the average time from diagnosis to death is 8 years.

Alzheimer's disease is the most common degenerative neurologic illness and the most common cause of cognitive impairment in adults; it currently affects more than 4 million people in the United States. (See *Theories about Alzheimer's disease*, page 144.) Early-onset Alzheimer's disease, which is rare, can affect adults ages 30 to 60. Usually, however, the disease affects people older than age 60.

Brain changes

After the patient's death, characteristic autopsy findings include loss of nerve cells and the presence of neurofibrillary tangles and amyloid plaques in the brain. These tangles and plaques disrupt transmission of nerve impulses and communication between neurons. Consequently, blood flow to affected brain areas decreases, and the brain atrophies. As the disease progresses, more brain areas are affected, with added symptoms corresponding to the affected areas. (See *Staging Alzheimer's disease*, pages 145 and 146.)

Several structural and chemical changes occur in the brain, especially in the hippocampus and the frontal and temporal lobes of the cerebral cortex. As neurons in the hippocampus and related structures are destroyed, short-term memory fails, and the patient's ability to perform familiar tasks declines. As neurons in the cerebral cortex are destroyed, the patient loses language skills and judgment, and emotions become increasingly labile. Eventually, the person becomes completely dependent and unresponsive.

Theories about Alzheimer's disease

No one knows what causes Alzheimer's disease or much about what raises the risk of developing it. Here are some theories.

Risk factors

The main risk factors for Alzheimer's disease seem to be age, family history, and the presence of the apolipoprotein E (apoE) allele on chromosome 19.

■ The likelihood of being diagnosed with Alzheimer's disease doubles for every 5 years of age beyond age 65.

■ People who have a first-degree relative diagnosed with Alzheimer's disease face a fourfold increase in the risk of developing the disease. This risk is even greater if the disease shows up in more than one generation.

■ ApoE is a protein that appears on the surface of cholesterol molecules and helps carry cholesterol throughout the body. It's also found in neurons of healthy brains and in amyloid plaques and neurofibrillary tangles. Carriers of the ApoE allele have have an increased risk of Alzheimer's disease; those with two copies of the gene have an even greater risk. However, this genetic pattern also occurs in people without Alzheimer's disease.

■ Other risk factors for Alzheimer's disease (and other dementias) include cerebral damage, hypertension, peripheral vascular disease, less education, and a history of traumatic brain injury.

Causes

Causes of Alzheimer's disease may include:

■ loss of neurotransmitter stimulation by choline acetyltransferase

■ a mutation for encoding an amyloid precursor protein

■ an alteration in apolipoprotein E

■ gene defects on chromosomes 14, 19, or 21 that promote clumping and precipitation of insoluble amyloid as plaques in the brain.

Disease stages

Alzheimer's disease has been classified in multiple ways, with some using a simple three-point scale and others listing up to seven stages based on symptoms and performance. However it's classified, Alzheimer's disease invariably leads to the patient's death and the need for palliative care.

Staging Alzheimer's disease

Although there's no standardized system for staging Alzheimer's disease, you can use these general categories.

Stage	Characteristics
Mild	▪ Trouble with word- or name-finding ▪ Trouble retaining names of new acquaintances ▪ Trouble retaining written material ▪ Misplaces or loses valuable objects ▪ Decreased ability to plan and carry out activities ▪ Some trouble maintaining social conversation ▪ Generally intact judgment ▪ Declining work skills
Moderate	▪ Inability to remember recent events and larger current events ▪ Trouble counting backward from 100 by 7s ▪ Decreased ability to handle finances ▪ Declining memory of personal history ▪ Trouble completing complex tasks ▪ Withdrawal in social situations ▪ Clouded judgment when complex issues arise ▪ Clear deficits in work skills
Moderately severe	▪ Inability to remember current address or telephone number but can remember own name and names of family and familiar people ▪ Trouble with simple arithmetic and reading ▪ Decreased ability to identify the date, season ▪ Decreased memory of recent personal history ▪ Needs help with simple tasks ▪ May respond inappropriately to social questions ▪ Impaired judgment about personal safety issues ▪ Unable to work ▪ Declining ability to dress appropriately to season or follow social conventions for eating in groups ▪ Early signs of personality changes possible
Severe	▪ Disoriented to place and time but usually can remember own name ▪ Possibly impaired sleep-wake cycle ▪ Declining interest in reading or former activities because of increasing confusion ▪ Inability to recall date or significant seasons or holidays, including birthday

(continued)

Staging Alzheimer's disease *(continued)*

Stage	Characteristics
Severe *(continued)*	■ Declining ability to recount personal history ■ Inability to carry out simple tasks, although may enjoy listening and watching ■ May forget family or caregiver names but recalls familiar faces ■ May make inappropriate judgments in familiar situations or may wander ■ Trouble with dressing, grooming, toileting, eating with utensils ■ Possible personality changes, such as suspicion, anxiety, delusions, anger ■ Possible start of urinary or fecal incontinence
End-stage	■ Disoriented to person, place, and time ■ No interest in former pastimes or ability to reason ■ Decreased evidence of awareness of surroundings ■ Forgets family and familiar faces ■ Inability to participate in daily activities ■ Inability to speak or very rarely speaks intelligibly ■ Has no judgment skills ■ Needs help with all activities of daily living, forgets how to swallow or chew food ■ Persistent personality changes that may affect caregiving ease ■ Incontinent at all times ■ Inability to walk, gradual inability to sit upright, becoming bedbound

Huntington's disease

Huntington's disease is a progressive, degenerative, inherited neurologic disease characterized by increasing dementia, speech problems, and choreiform (rapid, jerking, involuntary) movements. The disease was once called Huntington's chorea (from the Greek *khoreia*, which means "dance") because of the characteristic rhythmic, lurching gait that arises late in the disease.

This single-gene, autosomal dominant disease causes localized death of neurons in the basal ganglia. The genetic defect appears on chromosome 4 and involves an abnormally large number of the triplet DNA bases named CAG (cytosine-adenosine-guanine). The CAG triplet codes for the amino acid glutamine. When the protein *huntingtin* has a particularly long seg-

How Huntington's disease progresses

Stage	Psychosocial symptoms	Motor symptoms
Early	■ Irritability ■ Outbursts of rage alternating with euphoria ■ Depression ■ Emotional lability ■ Decreased ability to concentrate ■ Impulsiveness ■ Memory losses	■ Restlessness ■ Minor gait changes ■ Imbalance ■ Disturbed posture and positioning ■ Frequent falls ■ Protruding tongue ■ Slurred speech
Late	■ Severe memory deficits ■ Loss of cognitive skills ■ Disorientation to place and time ■ Confusion	■ Severely altered gait with irregular, uncontrollable movement, especially in distal extremities ■ Rhythmic shrugging of shoulders ■ Facial grimacing, including eyebrow raising and tongue protrusion ■ Dysphagia ■ Dysarthria ■ Impaired diaphragm movement

ment of glutamine, it forms aggregates in brain tissue, which may contribute to the neurodegeneration characteristic of Huntington's disease. CAG that repeats more than 39 times is reliably linked to development of the disease; indeed, the higher the number of triplet repeats, the earlier the onset of symptoms.

Although the exact pathogenesis is unclear, autopsies show a decrease in acetylcholine and gamma-aminobutyric acid in the basal ganglia. The acetylcholine deficit allows unopposed dopamine action, which causes excessive, uncontrolled movement. Psychological difficulties may precede choreiform movements.

Disease progression

After symptoms begin, Huntington's disease progresses slowly over 10 to 25 years. Cells are destroyed in the caudate nucleus and putamen, areas of the striatum located in the basal ganglia. Other areas of the brain, such as the frontal lobes, may atrophy as well. (See *How Huntington's disease progresses.*)

Motor symptoms usually parallel personality and mood changes. Initially, the patient may describe feeling restless or fidgety. Then, choreiform movements progressively worsen, starting in the face and arms and eventually involving the entire body. Environmental stimuli and emotional stress may aggravate the symptoms; they may stop when the patient is sleeping. The constant movements and increasing trouble swallowing contribute to weight loss and eventual cachexia. Breathing becomes impaired because the diaphragm can't move effectively. Prognosis is poor in the late stages of disease, with inevitable debilitation, total dependence, and dementia.

 LIFESPAN Although carriers of the Huntington's disease genetic defect can be identified through genetic testing, many at-risk people choose not to be tested because the results would come too late. Because symptoms typically don't start until age 30 to 40, many people already have passed the gene to their children by the time they consider testing. In fact, it's common for several family members to develop the disease.

The psychological impact of Huntington's disease can be devastating to patients and their families, not only from feelings of guilt for passing on the disease, but also from the overwhelming long-term care needs of those affected. Providing palliative care for patients with Huntington's disease and their families presents many substantial challenges. Massive physiologic and psychosocial problems result from the progressive and eventually debilitating nature of the disease. Not only will the patient need a great deal of direct care, but the family will need a great deal of help as well. Having an experienced multidisciplinary care team is essential in helping the patient and family cope with this difficult disease.

End-stage neurologic disease

Because ALS, Alzheimer's disease, and Huntington's disease are invariably terminal, and because patients gradually lose their ability to communicate their wishes, it's critical that your patient complete a living will — in which he specifies the treatments he does and doesn't want — while he's still able. Carefully review the typical course of the patient's disease, and discuss his desire for such treatments as gastrostomy tube placement, ventilatory assistance, and invasive procedures used to prolong life.

Also, urge the patient to designate someone as his health care power of attorney. Explain that doing so establishes the legal right of that person to make health care decisions for the patient when he's no longer able. Make sure his advance directives are documented properly, and give a copy to his primary care provider. Involve the patient's family in this discussion so they're better able to support his wishes. If the patient resists making advance directives, urge him to at least talk with loved ones about these critical decisions.

Starting palliative care

Patients with dementia are at particular risk for receiving poor end-of-life care, in part because it's so difficult to establish a relatively reliable estimate of when life expectancy has reached 6 months — a requirement for entering hospice care. Perhaps this is why fewer than 2% of hospice patients have a primary diagnosis of dementia. Use a performance status scale to estimate the six-month window. On most scales, a score of 30% or less is often interpreted as a life expectancy that's less than 6 months.

Whether the patient's life expectancy is clear or not, advancing disease places a great burden on caregivers as they struggle to provide supportive end-of-life care for the patient. A palliative care team with an individualized, collaborative approach provides immeasurable assistance; earlier interventions delivered before the disease advanced are more helpful than simply a late referral for hospice care. (See *Hospice or palliative care?*, page 150.) Palliative care maintains quality of life for the patient and his family.

Home health nursing, social work, and physical, occupational, speech, and respiratory therapy are major supportive and rehabilitative resources in palliative care. Rehabilitative care is essential to help the patient adjust to the progressive decline in physical function. These health care professionals can teach alternative ways of performing activities of daily living based on the patient's individual symptoms and disease stage. Geriatric psychiatrists can be helpful in implementing palliative care and hospice and they remain an important part of the care once it is in place.

Managing symptoms

Once the patient and family have entered palliative or hospice care, many symptoms of terminal neurologic disease will need to be addressed and managed. Offering both drug and nondrug approaches can give additional control to patients and their families in managing symptoms. Certainly, each patient will have a unique set of symptoms and difficulties. However, symptoms common to ALS, Alzheimer's disease, and Huntington's disease include pain, anxiety, depression, dysphagia, and asthenia.

Pain

Many patients with advancing dementia don't have the verbal or cognitive skills to report their pain. Consequently, identifying and assessing pain can be very challenging. Plus, the patient's anxiety, depression, or hostility can distract you from recognizing the pain that he may be experiencing.

If the patient has a known source of pain from a preexisting illness, caregivers should continue to give whatever drugs or treatments have proved helpful to the patient. Also, if the patient can't communicate clearly, watch for nonverbal cues to his pain level, such as grimacing, bracing, rubbing, restlessness, or agitation.

EXPERT INSIGHTS

Hospice or palliative care?

When I told a colleague that I was interested in specializing in hospice, she said, "It's not called hospice anymore. You mean palliative care." Am I confusing these terms? — K.H., N.C.

Although some people use the terms "hospice" and "palliative care" interchangeably, they're not the same. Palliative care is the broader term; hospice care is one of the programs within the scope of palliative care.

Besides physical care, palliative care can include counseling, social support, spiritual guidance, and even financial assistance. The World Health Organization proposes that palliative care have these characteristics:

■ recognition that cure or long-term control isn't possible
■ concern with the quality rather than the quantity of life
■ treatment of troublesome and distressing symptoms with the primary or sole aim of keeping the patient as comfortable as possible.

You don't see the words "terminal" or "dying" because the principles and practices of true palliative care should be employed before the final days or weeks of life. I've always felt that palliative care begins as soon as the patient needs it.

Let's say your 70-year-old patient is diagnosed with chronic myelogenous leukemia. Before he's discharged, his oncologist should discuss anticipated treatment outcomes. The physician needs to frankly explain that, although the disease isn't curable, he'll make every effort to prevent pain and manage other symptoms.

This patient probably wouldn't choose hospice now because he can expect to live a few more years. However, he could benefit from palliative care in the form of social, emotional, and financial support, if he chooses. At some point he may say, "I'm finished with all of this and just want to be made comfortable, with no more trips to the hospital." Then hospice steps in.

Regardless of the differences, hospice and palliative care have one thing in common: a staff committed to helping patients live and die with dignity. No matter which choice you make, you're sure to fit in.

— JOY UFEMA, RN, MS

NSAIDs are the first line of drug treatments for musculoskeletal pain. If these are ineffective, then short-acting, immediate-release morphine may be used in liquid or dissolvable tablet form to relieve acute pain. For patients with an identifiable source of pain, longer acting drugs such as a fentanyl (Duragesic) patch or sustained-release morphine may be used.

Patients who have spasticity and fasciculations are prone to muscle cramping, which can be very painful. Drugs that can help manage these problems include:

■ baclofen (Lioresal)
■ carbamazepine (Tegretol)
■ phenytoin (Dilantin)
■ quinine sulfate
■ magnesium
■ verapamil (Calan)
■ vitamin E.

You'll have to adjust each of these drugs to the patient's comfort, not with the goal of ending the visible evidence of spasticity. Keep in mind that some degree of spasticity is important in allowing the patient to remain mobile.

Immobility and joint contractures can be problems for patients with ALS and Alzheimer's disease, and both can be painful. Massage can help reduce muscle pain, and frequent repositioning and passive range-of-motion exercises can help prevent contractures and pain.

No matter what the origin of the patient's pain, your goal is to keep the patient comfortable while maintaining his ability to interact with loved ones.

Anxiety

Common to all dying patients and their families, anxiety about impending death can be overwhelming. Questions about what will happen, what it will feel like, and what the family should do, are understandably common sources of anxiety for the patient and family members. You and other members of the multidisciplinary team can have a soothing effect on anxiety by addressing the patient's and family's concerns and answering their questions as honestly and openly as you can.

For persistent anxiety, psychosocial support and psychotherapy are appropriate. A neuropsychologist can be instrumental in addressing psychosocial concerns. If available, one-on-one sessions can help to alleviate many sources of anxiety.

If the patient needs drug therapy to help ease anxiety, benzodiazepines usually are the first choice. Use these drugs cautiously, however, because accumulation and combination therapy can lead to delirium. First-line therapy typically includes a short-acting benzodiazepine, such as lorazepam (Ativan) or oxazepam (Serax). If anxiety persists, the patient may need a more powerful tranquilizer, such as haloperidol (Haldol). Monitor the patient closely when starting such drugs.

Nondrug treatments for anxiety include acupuncture, massage, and guided imagery with relaxation therapy.

Depression

Understandably, diseases such as ALS, Alzheimer's disease, and Huntington's disease can leave patients and families feeling helpless, hopeless, and depressed. Sadness usually responds to supportive interventions; however, depression is a more persistent state marked by greater cognitive impairment and should be treated aggressively. Suspect depression if the patient has persistent episodes of intense sadness, anhedonia, and depressive symptoms for more than a few days or weeks.

If the patient has sleep disruption along with depression, a tricyclic antidepressant given at bedtime may be the most effective treatment. A selective serotonin reuptake inhibitor (SSRI) or a serotonin and norepinephrine reuptake inhibitor (SNRI) will cause less daytime drowsiness but may take weeks to reach a therapeutic effect.

A psychostimulant may offer a safe way to improve energy, concentration, and mood while an SSRI or SNRI takes effect and also may counteract the sedating effects of opioids. Dextroamphetamine (Dexedrine), methylphenidate (Ritalin), and modafinil (Provigil) have a fast rate and a short duration of action. These drugs can greatly improve the quality of the patient's last few months of life.

Dysphagia

An inability to chew or swallow safely can be issues for patients with any of these neurologic diseases. When symptoms begin, it may be helpful to change the patient's diet to soft foods and thickened liquids. Also, consider having a speech therapist work with the patient and family to teach ways to improve swallowing and safety while eating.

 ALERT For the ALS patient in particular, a percutaneous endoscopic gastrostomy (PEG) tube can maintain nutrition and weight for a time. However, the decision to place a PEG tube brings with it the need to decide when the tube feedings are no longer useful and may, in fact, be harmful to the patient. When food can no longer be effectively translated into nutrients by the gut and kidneys, overfeeding and discomfort can result. Plus, a PEG tube doesn't reduce the risk of aspiration, leaving these patients vulnerable to pneumonia.

Asthenia

Asthenia, or profound tiredness after a usual or minimal effort, is a common symptom in dying patients. They may describe it as generalized weakness. To treat it, start by determining whether it has any specific causes. Examples include depression, infection, and anemia. Also, consult physical and occupational therapists about energy conservation techniques and modifications to activities of daily living.

Special issues in amyotrophic lateral sclerosis

ALS patients experience some unique symptoms that require special care at the end of life. (See *Special care issues in amyotrophic lateral sclerosis,* page 154.) A multidisciplinary approach is helpful in addressing these needs.

Preparing the patient and family for the progressive losses caused by ALS can be a powerful form of assistance. For instance, when the physician determines that the patient will soon lose his ability to speak, the speech and physical therapist can work with the patient and family to learn alternative methods of communication, such as blinking. Such interventions can help to alleviate fear and anxiety, strengthen the patient's and family's psychological and physical adaptation, and help create a more peaceful dying process.

Special issues in Alzheimer's disease

Certain problems arise more often in patients with Alzheimer's disease than in those with other neurologic diseases, and they warrant attentive palliative care. One such problem is how to maintain human contact with the patient as dementia increases. Providing social support and contact involves talking to a patient with dementia, even if you do most of the talking. One-on-one contact or simulated presence therapy, in which the patient views or listens to taped recordings of loved ones, can be helpful for the Alzheimer's patient. Pet therapy, massage therapy, and doll therapy have also been used to comfort the patient with Alzheimer's and may be an effective mechanism for social contact with nonverbal patients who have advanced dementia.

Maintaining comfortable and consistent surroundings for the person with advanced Alzheimer's disease is important in retaining as much cognitive capacity as possible. It's also important to provide appropriate amounts of stimulation, which can be addressed through passive and active engagement activities. Passive engagement activities include music, aromatherapy, and touch therapy. Active engagement usually is offered in the form of structured activities, including group and individual activities such as modified sewing, writing together, reading, sorting, or walking.

Behavior problems Agitation, aggression, irritability, and restlessness are common in patients with dementia. Before starting drug treatment for these behavioral symptoms, identify and modify all external factors that could be responsible, such as changes in environment or reference person, confrontations with caregivers, or too much or too little external stimuli. Also consider the effect of other illnesses and adverse drug effects. If behavioral problems persist after correcting all external causes, prioritize the patient's problems and begin addressing them with targeted drug therapy. Aim for monotherapy if possible, introducing one drug at a time and adjusting that drug before changing or adding a new one. As a rule, drug therapy

COMFORT & CARE

Special care issues in amyotrophic lateral sclerosis

Issue	Cause	Treatment
Drooling	Bulbar dysfunction	■ Amitriptyline at bedtime can help but increases gastroesophageal reflux and constipation. ■ Glycopyrrolate (Robinul) and hyoscamine (Levsin drops) minimize the effect and risk of cognitive failure. ■ Transdermal scopolamine helps compliance because the patch only needs changed every 3 days.
Dyspnea and hypoventilation	Weakened diaphragm and accessory respiratory muscles	■ Oxygen rarely is used because it may worsen hypoventilation and cause hypercapnia. ■ Bilevel positive airway pressure (known as BiPAP) is best initially, starting intermittently or during sleep. ■ Invasive ventilation is a choice that should be addressed in the patient's advance directives. ■ During terminal care, lorazepam (Ativan) and morphine may be given for comfort and to reduce anxiety-related dyspnea.
Dysarthria	Weakened muscles of articulation	■ Alphabet charts and computer technology are helpful while the patient retains voluntary muscle movement. ■ Coded blinking can be taught to patients and caregivers for use at end stages.
Insomnia or interrupted sleep	Immobility, muscle cramping, respiratory insufficiency, anxiety, and depression	■ BiPAP will help if desaturation is occurring. ■ Use sleeping aids cautiously if BiPAP isn't in place. ■ Antidepressants or anxiolytics may be helpful.

should start at low doses and be increased slowly. In general, drugs with no or few adverse anticholinergic effects are preferred.

Low-dose classical neuroleptics, such as haloperidol or thioridazine, are effective for behavioral symptoms and can be especially helpful if the patient also has hallucinations or delusions.

 ALERT Avoid giving benzodiazepines because they can worsen cognitive function and may cause paradoxical reactions, such as increased confusion and agitation.

Depression and obsession Depression or depressive and obsessive components are common in neurocognitive diseases. In general, avoid drugs with anticholinergic effects, such as tricyclic antidepressants. Instead, use an SSRI such as citalopram (Celexa) or sertraline (Zoloft). Other central nervous system agents, such as fluvoxamine (Luvox), may have beneficial effects as well. These drugs can improve depressive symptoms, disinhibition, and compulsions in patients with frontotemporal dementia. Mood fluctuations and emotional lability or bursts may respond to mood stabilizers such as carbamazepine (Tegretol) and sodium valproate (Depakote).

Sleep disturbance Many patients with Alzheimer's disease develop sleep disturbances—including trouble falling asleep, frequent waking, night wandering, and changes in diurnal rhythms, including sundowning. Drugs that may improve insomnia include:
■ the sedative antidepressant trazodone (Tranxene)
■ the non-benzodiazepine hypnotic zolpidem (Ambien)
■ low-dose classical neuroleptics such as haloperidol (Haldol) and thioridazine (Mellaril)
■ atypical neuroleptics, such as clozapine (Clozaril), olanzapine (Zyprexa) or risperidone (Risperdal)
■ chloral hydrate.

Benzodiazepines should be the last resort and should be used only for short-term treatment. If the patient also has depression, treating it can also improve sleep.

Psychosis Such psychotic symptoms as visual or auditory hallucinations, delusions, and visual or auditory misperceptions can at times be more disturbing to the family than the patient's cognitive deficits. Treating these symptoms may bring major relief to caregivers as well as to the patient. Classic neuroleptics such as haloperidol improve these symptoms, as well as atypical neuroleptics such as clozapine, olanzapine, or risperidone. Other drugs, such as carbamazepine, sodium valproate, buspirone (BuSpar), and propranolol (Inderal), may be used to treat agitation.

11 | **Patients with pulmonary disease**

The pulmonary disorders most likely to lead to end-of-life care—other than lung cancer, which is addressed in Chapter 8—are chronic obstructive pulmonary disease, other restrictive lung diseases, and cystic fibrosis.

Chronic obstructive pulmonary disease

Chronic obstructive pulmonary disease (COPD) is a slowly progressive disorder that affects more than 14 million Americans. About 24 million have impaired lung function, suggesting that COPD is even more common than we think. COPD is the fourth leading cause of death in the United States.

COPD includes two disorders that obstruct air movement into and out of the lungs: emphysema and chronic bronchitis. The patient may have one or both disorders. Asthma is no longer considered a form of COPD. It's now defined as a mainly reversible airflow disorder caused by airway inflammation. However, when severe, asthma may cause airway obstruction and lead to serious disability. (See *Comparing emphysema, chronic bronchitis, and asthma*, pages 158 and 159.) COPD can be categorized based on severity.

Emphysema
The American Thoracic Society defines emphysema as permanent enlargement of the distal airspaces, destruction of their walls, and no obvious fibrosis. Over time, air space becomes deadened with little or no participation in blood–gas exchange. Dyspnea is a hallmark sign of this disorder. About 2 million Americans have this disease; almost 1 million have both chronic bronchitis and emphysema.

Chronic bronchitis

Chronic bronchitis involves inflammation of the bronchi (the main passages in the lungs), excessive bronchial mucus production, and a chronic productive cough. Increased mucus volume and consistency impairs mucociliary function in the bronchioles and distal airways. As mucus and inflammation thicken bronchial passages, the risk of infection also increases.

In end-stage chronic bronchitis, the patient may have severe exacerbations, reduced alveolar ventilation, abnormal ventilation-perfusion, hypoxemia (PaO_2 < 50% to 60%), increasing levels of $PaCO_2$, and polycythemia (compensation for decreased PaO_2).

Management

Treatment and supportive measures for patients with COPD include monitoring of diagnostic criteria and patient education. Because COPD progresses slowly, ongoing monitoring can help you detect changes early and intervene promptly. Monitoring may include:

- arterial blood gas measurements
- assessment of patient's symptoms and feelings about quality of life
- chest X-rays
- laboratory tests, such as a complete blood count, especially for hemoglobin level and hematocrit to monitor oxygenation status
- pulmonary function tests
- pulmonary rehabilitation
- pulse oximetry.

Urge the patient to avoid smoke and to stop smoking if applicable. Clearly, this task may be very difficult for a patient who has already tried repeatedly to stop smoking. Suggest that the patient also avoid other triggers that could cause COPD to flare up, such as pollution, chemicals, noxious fumes, and infections—although doing so may increase the patient's sense of isolation and limitation.

Also, teach the patient about the disease process, symptom management, and drug therapy to help manage COPD symptoms. Some patients medically qualify for lung volume reduction surgery, which improves oxygenation and quality of life for about 4 years after it's performed. Recommend annual flu vaccination and regular vaccination against pneumococcal pneumonia.

Drug therapy

The goal of drug therapy is to decrease inflammation in the distal bronchioles and alveoli, aid bronchodilation, decrease mucus production, and treat infection if needed. Drug therapy can't stop changes that have already occurred in the lung tissue, but it can relieve some symptoms.

Comparing emphysema, chronic bronchitis, and asthma

Disease	Causes and pathophysiology
Emphysema ■ Destruction of alveolar walls causes irreversible enlargement of air spaces distal to terminal bronchioles and decreased elastic recoil of lungs. ■ *Prognosis:* Most common cause of death from respiratory disease in the United States.	■ Cigarette smoking and congenital deficiency of alpha$_1$-antitrypsin. ■ Recurrent inflammation and release of proteolytic enzymes from lung cells damages and ultimately destroys bronchiolar and alveolar walls. Loss of supporting lung structure results in decreased elastic recoil and airway collapse on expiration. Destruction of alveolar walls decreases surface area for gas exchange.
Chronic bronchitis ■ Patient has excessive mucus production and productive cough for at least 3 months yearly for 2 consecutive years. ■ *Prognosis:* Significant airway obstruction possible but uncommon.	■ Severity depends on amount and duration of smoking; respiratory infection worsens symptoms. ■ Hypertrophy and hyperplasia of bronchial mucous glands, increased goblet cells, damage to cilia, squamous metaplasia of columnar epithelium, and chronic leukocytic and lymphocytic infiltration of bronchial walls; widespread inflammation, distortion, narrowing of airways, and mucus in the airways produce resistance in small airways and cause severe ventilation-perfusion imbalance.
Asthma ■ Bronchial reactivity to many stimuli is increased, which produces episodic bronchospasm, airway obstruction, and airway inflammation. ■ Childhood onset usually related to certain allergens. Adult onset usually without distinct allergies. ■ Status asthmaticus is an acute attack with severe bronchospasm that doesn't respond to broncho-dilator therapy. ■ *Prognosis:* With childhood onset, usually no adult symptoms; with adult onset, usually persistent disease and occasional severe attacks.	■ Reversible airway inflammation usually occurs in response to an allergen. Swelling of membranes, bronchoconstriction, and production of mucus obstruct airways. Activated mast cells release chemical mediators, including histamine, bradykinin, prostaglandins, and leukotrienes, which perpetuate the inflammatory response. ■ Upper airway infection, exercise, anxiety and, rarely, coughing or laughing can cause an asthma attack; nocturnal flare-ups are common. Paroxysmal airway obstruction with nasal polyps may occur in response to aspirin or indomethacin ingestion. Airway obstruction may result from spasm of bronchial smooth muscle that narrows airways; inflammatory edema of the bronchial wall, and thickening of tenacious mucoid secretions, particularly in status asthmaticus.

Clinical features

■ Insidious onset, with dyspnea the main symptom.
■ *Other signs and symptoms of long-term disease:* anorexia, weight loss, malaise, barrel chest, use of accessory muscles of respiration, prolonged expiratory period with grunting, pursed-lip breathing, and tachypnea.
■ *Complications:* recurrent respiratory tract infections, cor pulmonale, and respiratory failure.

■ Insidious onset, with productive cough and exertional dyspnea the main symptoms.
■ *Other signs:* upper respiratory infections with increased sputum production and worsening dyspnea, which take progressively longer to resolve; copious sputum (gray, white, or yellow); weight gain from edema; cyanosis; tachypnea; wheezing; prolonged expiratory time; and use of accessory muscles of respiration.
■ *Complications:* recurrent respiratory tract infections, cor pulmonale, and polycythemia.

■ History of intermittent attacks of dyspnea and wheezing.
■ Mild wheezing progresses to severe dyspnea, audible wheezing, chest tightness (a feeling of not being able to breathe), and cough that produces thick mucus.
■ *Other signs:* prolonged expiration, intercostal and supraclavicular retraction on inspiration, use of accessory muscles of respiration, flaring nostrils, tachypnea, tachycardia, perspiration, and flushing; patients usually have symptoms of eczema and allergic rhinitis (hay fever).
■ *Complications:* status asthmaticus, which can progress to respiratory failure if not treated promptly.

Drugs for chronic obstructive pulmonary disease

Drug	Actions	Adverse effects
Beta₂ agonists		
albuterol (Proventil), metaproterenol (Alupent), salmeterol (Serevent)	Acts on beta₂ receptors to relax smooth muscles in the bronchial tree	Heartburn, hypokalemia, muscle tremors and cramps, nausea, tachycardia, vomiting
Anticholinergics		
ipratropium (Atrovent), tiotropium (Spiriva)	Blocks acetylcholine action at parasympathetic sites in bronchial smooth muscle	Dizziness, dry mouth, fatigue, headache, nervousness
Leukotriene inhibitors		
montelukast (Singulair), zafirlukast (Accolate)	Blocks leukotrienes, which mediate inflammation	Headache, nausea, prolonged warfarin (Coumadin) action
Methylxanthines		
theophylline (Theo-Dur), aminophylline (Truphylline)	Dilates the bronchial tree by increasing tissue levels of cyclic adenosine monophosphate	Dizziness, gastric upset, nausea, nervousness, palpitations, possible toxicity, tachycardia, vomiting
Mucolytics		
acetylcysteine (Mucomyst), dornase alfa (Pulmozyme)	Thins viscous secretions by breaking bonds between large proteins	Bronchospasm, irritation of tracheal and bronchial tracts, nausea, stomatitis, vomiting
Corticosteroids		
beclomethasone (Vanceril), methylprednisolone (Solu-Medrol), prednisone (Deltasone)	Reduces inflammatory response in bronchial walls by suppressing the action of white blood cells and immune system	Adrenal suppression (high doses), cough, decreased resistance to infection, dysphoria, fragile skin, heart failure, hyperglycemia, hypertension, oral thrush, peptic ulcer

Bronchodilators, (including beta$_2$ agonists, anticholinergics, and methylxanthines), leukotriene inhibitors, mucolytics, and corticosteroids are used most often. (See *Drugs for chronic obstructive pulmonary disease.*)

Use of corticosteroids is limited in patients with COPD but no asthma. Acute exacerbations of COPD do respond to short courses of corticosteroids, but long-term use doesn't seem to be effective in reducing exacerbations or improving prognosis.

Antibiotics may be given for infection as a comfort measure. In end-stage disease, however, the patient may choose to stop antibiotic treatment. Make sure to address this issue with any severely impaired patient with a decreasing quality of life and limited improvement from previous antibiotic therapy.

Oxygen therapy

Oxygen corrects the hypoxemia that occurs throughout the disease. The lungs try to compensate for decreased compliance caused by hyperventilation. It was once thought that giving more than 2 L/ minute of oxygen would diminish the patient's respiratory drive. It's now known that patients should be given enough oxygen to keep the O$_2$ saturation level at 90% or above. Treating the hypoxia increases comfort and quality of life without significantly affecting the lungs' compensatory drive.

Initially, oxygen may be used intermittently during exercise and sleep when oxygen saturation falls below 89%. Continuous oxygen therapy usually isn't needed until the disease is very severe. Oxygen therapy prolongs life and may improve the patient's mental outlook. Use it in any patient who wants it and reports improvement — but consider not using it even in end-stage disease if the patient is more comfortable without it. (See *Taking off the mask,* pages 162 and 163.)

End-of-life care

Because COPD symptoms progress so slowly, it can be tough to tell when the disease has reached its final stages. By assessing the patient regularly, you can help to control such common symptoms as dyspnea, depression, anxiety, and others.

Dyspnea

As COPD progresses, functioning lung tissue decreases and lung compliance worsens — usually leading to dyspnea. Dyspnea is a subjective symptom that the person may describe as an awareness of breathing and increasing trouble doing so. Physical signs that suggest dyspnea include:
- labored breathing

EXPERT INSIGHTS

Taking off the mask

I read a column of yours in which you said you removed the oxygen mask from a dying patient's face because he wasn't struggling to breathe. When I mentioned this to one of my nursing colleagues, she said depriving a patient of supplemental oxygen is unacceptable because it would hasten his death. Can you explain your thinking?
— N.W., Texas

When a patient is in the final stages of illness and the goal is comfort care, I believe oxygen should be given only rarely because it may prolong the dying process. Oxygen typically isn't needed for comfort. Morphine and lorazepam (Ativan) will do an excellent job of keeping a dying patient comfortable by sedating her and preventing respiratory failure.

I learned about this from an intensivist who was weaning a dying patient from a ventilator. When writing orders, he deliberately withheld an order for oxygen. He did, however, order a morphine infusion "to be titrated for comfort." This gave the nurses plenty of leeway to use their judgment if the patient began laboring to breathe.

A few weeks ago, I worked with a 62-year-old woman actively dying of lung cancer. She was comatose and appeared quite comfortable on 4 mg of morphine hourly. Her two older sisters were camped at the bedside, sharing treasured moments.

The patient was receiving 50% oxygen via a venturi mask. Wondering if she really needed the oxygen, I gently examined her and found that her hands and feet were warm and pink, without signs of cyanosis. Her respirations were 6 per minute, deep and even.

- shortness of breath at rest or with exertion
- increased respiratory rate (more than 24 breaths per minute)
- increased respiratory effort
- altered lung sounds.

In later stages of COPD, you may notice the patient using accessory muscles of respiration, or he may complain of pain with breathing.

During your assessment, find out whether the patient has started any new drugs, increased or decreased a dosage, changed his activity level, or noticed any new symptoms (such as hemoptysis, fever, or worsening pain).

I got the visitors some lunch, then returned 4 hours later. Reassessing the patient, I found her condition unchanged. Noticing the sisters were preparing to spend the night, I asked them how long the patient had been in the hospital.

"Three days," the older one replied. "She was just like this at home, except without a mask. She just had those little prongs in her nose."

The other sister smiled. "Helen was always vain about her looks. She wouldn't like wearing a mask."

I asked the women to join me in the hall.

"Your sister is in a deep coma and appears quite comfortable," I said. "I don't think the oxygen is doing anything to help her, and it may be prolonging the dying process. You need to hear me clearly when I say I'm not trying to hurry her along to die sooner. I just want you to have the information. Do you think she's waiting to complete any unfinished business before she dies?"

They said no in unison.

"We've been telling her that it's okay to go, that we'll be all right, but she's not going," said one.

"Do you want the mask to come off?" I asked.

"We'll talk with her son when he comes in tonight," said the other sister. "We understand what you're telling us, and we both agree."

In the end, the family decided against removing the mask; I don't know why. Perhaps Helen's son had some unfinished business of his own. But it was important to tell the family about the implications of oxygen therapy so they could make an informed decision.

In my book, this is true palliative care.

— *JOY UFEMA, RN, MS*

Changes in these areas may suggest a specific cause for the patient's dyspnea, such as infection, and warrant further evaluation or treatment.

One of the most important goals in caring for a patient with end-stage COPD is to maintain his comfort level by treating the primary cause or causes of dyspnea while providing emotional support and education. Oxygen therapy may be helpful. Certain nondrug therapies also may help decrease dyspnea or the anxiety that commonly accompanies it. (See *Nondrug methods to relieve dyspnea*, page 164.) Opioids may help as well; they're highly effective in relieving dyspnea and cough. In fact, opioids are

COMFORT & CARE

Nondrug methods to relieve dyspnea

- Acupuncture
- Cool air flowing over the head and chest (fan, air conditioner, open window)
- Breathing exercises, such as pursed-lip breathing

- Hypnosis
- Massage
- Presence of a calm person
- Relaxation therapy
- Sight of other people

standard treatment for patients nearing death. Dyspnea may decrease as the ventilatory drive decreases.

Depression and anxiety

About half of patients with COPD develop symptoms of depression and anxiety. Stay alert for this development, and use a standardized tool to help assess the patient's condition. Common tools include the Beck Depression Inventory, Geriatric Depression Scale, Zung Depression Scale, and Hamilton Anxiety Rating Scale.

Drug therapy may help relieve the patient's depression or anxiety, but you'll need to make sure the drug chosen doesn't cause respiratory depression. The most common choice for treating depression in patients with COPD is a selective serotonin reuptake inhibitor. These drugs tend to have fewer adverse effects than tricyclic antidepressants. Nortriptyline (Pamelor), buspirone (BuSpar), and sertraline (Zoloft) have all been useful to many patients with anxiety or anxiety with a depressive component.

Cognitive behavior therapy, spiritual interventions, distraction, and relaxation techniques also may be useful for decreasing anxiety and depression in some patients.

Other symptoms

Other common symptoms of end-stage COPD include drowsiness from CO_2 retention and edema from right ventricular failure. If the patient has cardiac involvement, drugs can be added to decrease edema and cardiac workload. Low blood pressure or orthostatic hypotension may result from these treatments; teach the patient how to change positions safely.

Headaches and sleep apnea may arise in some patients. Head-aches can be treated with cool compresses and acetaminophen. In general, try to avoid nonsteroidal anti-inflammatory drugs because of the risk of increased edema.

For sleep apnea, a continuous positive airway pressure (CPAP) device used nasally may help. The CPAP provides extra air pressure to help keep the alveoli from compressing fully, thus reducing the work of breathing.

Restrictive lung disease

Restrictive lung diseases are disorders that affect lung volume and lung or chest-wall compliance. As a result, the overall lung capacity and ability of the lungs to participate in gas exchange is reduced. Restrictive lung diseases may be either intrapulmonary and extrapulmonary. (See *Causes of restrictive lung disease*.)

Assessment

Symptoms of restrictive lung disease vary with the cause. Most patients have shallow, rapid breathing and shortness of breath with exertion that later progresses to fatigue of the respiratory muscles, hypoxemia, and in-creased carbon dioxide levels.

Causes of restrictive lung disease

Restrictive lung disease may have an intrapulmonary or extrapul-monary cause. Here are some examples of each.

Intrapulmonary causes
- Atelectasis
- Neoplasm
- Pneumonia
- Pulmonary fibrosis
- Sarcoidosis
- Surgical lung resection

Extrapulmonary causes
- Amyotrophic lateral sclerosis
- Congenital wall deformities
- Excessive obesity
- Head or spinal cord injury
- Muscular dystrophy
- Myasthenia gravis
- Pleural effusion
- Sleep disorders

Pulmonary function testing is used to examine the degree of lung impairment. If total lung capacity is less than 80% of expected, the patient is diagnosed with the disorder. Chest X-rays, neurologic dysfunction testing (such as electromyography), immunologic testing, and arterial blood gas measurements are also used to rule out other potential causes for restrictive lung disease.

Management

Treatment depends on the specific cause of the disease. Oxygen may be needed to correct altered gas exchange. Priority nursing goals include:
- maintaining a patent airway
- providing adequate oxygenation based on patient need
- helping the patient maintain activities of daily living and physical function.

End stages of restrictive lung disease develop when hypoxemia becomes severe and less responsive to therapy. Cor pulmonale, pulmonary hypertension, and respiratory failure occur late in the disease.

End-of-life care

Palliative care for these patients involves treatments to reduce the effects of the underlying condition as well as supportive measures for cardiovascular effects. Issues in end-of-life care are similar to those in COPD.

Cystic fibrosis

Cystic fibrosis (CF) is a chronic multisystem genetic disorder affecting the exocrine glands. It's the second most common inherited disease of childhood in the United States, after sickle cell disease. CF is an autosomal recessive trait. If both parents carry the gene, each of their children has a 25% chance of developing the disease. Cystic fibrosis occurs in 1 of 4,000 births in white children. The disease is less common among blacks, Hispanics, and Asians. In the United States, about 80% of CF patients are diagnosed before age 18. However, diagnosis after age 18 is becoming more common.

Normally, the exocrine glands produce mucus in the bronchioles, small intestine, and bile and pancreatic ducts. In CF, the mucus produced is thick and obstructs the passageways of the organs. The average age of death for patients with cystic fibrosis is 33, although improvements in care have dramatically increased the life expectancy in both children and younger adults.

Symptoms and complications of cystic fibrosis

Patients with cystic fibrosis may develop various symptoms and complications, such as those listed here. Lung involvement is common, and liver involvement occurs in about 6% of patients. The severity of the disease also varies, affecting lifespan.

Symptoms
- Excessive appetite but poor weight gain
- Greasy, bulky stools
- Persistent coughing, at times with phlegm
- Skin that tastes very salty
- Wheezing, shortness of breath

Complications
- Diabetes
- Malnutrition from decreased digestive enzymes
- Osteoporosis
- Permanent liver damage from blocked bile duct
- Recurrent lung infections

Assessment

The symptoms of CF vary according to the main body system affected. Symptom severity increases over the course of the disease. (See *Symptoms and complications of cystic fibrosis.*)

Often, the first symptom of CF is meconium ileus, which is diagnostic for the disease. Otherwise, early detection of CF can be difficult based on symptoms alone because of the wide range of systems that may be affected and the relatively nonspecific nature of symptoms. Screening protocols have been developed to help detect CF as early as possible, allowing for early intervention and overall improvement of patient quality of life.

Prenatal screening for CF can be done by DNA analysis of amniotic fluid. Siblings of children with CF can be screened as carriers of the disease through DNA analysis via buccal smear or blood sample as well.

Newborns are tested after confirmation of bulky, greasy stools, poor growth rate, and frequent respiratory illnesses such as colds, bronchitis, and pneumonia. The sweat test is another diagnostic indicator used in CF. This test measures the amount of sodium and chloride in a sweat sample and is very reliable. Often performed twice to ensure accuracy, results showing a chloride level greater than 60 mEq/L are considered diagnostic.

Management

Treatment for CF is aimed at preventing respiratory infections, maintaining nutritional status, and providing emotional support. Treatment of respiratory infections at the earliest sign is crucial. Percussion and postural drainage help loosen and mobilize secretions. Children affected by CF should receive routine childhood immunizations as recommended by the American Academy of Pediatrics.

Drugs, such as mucolytic agents, anti-inflammatories, bronchodilators, oxygen, and antibiotics are routinely used in treating CF based on symptoms and patient need. Nutritional support and consultation with a dietitian are also suggested for CF patients because of their increased metabolism and related digestive problems.

Additional care for patients with CF includes interventions similar to those needed for other pulmonary diseases, such as these:

■ Maintain a patent airway and oxygenation.
■ Prevent infection.
■ Promote exercise and nutrition for growth.
■ Teach the patient and family about the disease.
■ Arrange for home care when needed.

Also, keep in mind the importance of emotional support for patients and families coping with a serious chronic illness. Refer them for counseling if needed. Encourage discussion of the child's needs and care with school personnel to help ensure compatible care at school and at home. Help parents learn how to foster independence in their child. Also, refer them to appropriate support groups and community resources, such as the American Lung Association, the Cystic Fibrosis Foundation, and other illness-specific organizations.

End-of-life care

Children with CF or other severe pulmonary disorders are often cared for in the home. The patient's physician and others on the care team should provide honest, clear information about the course of the disease, its treatment, and its prognosis. This information may need to be reinforced at various times.

The palliative care team may play an important role in assisting patients and families through the stages of the illness. When aggressive treatment is no longer feasible, the team can then assist in shifting the focus to a comfortable time of life before death. Parents in particular may need the extra support and ongoing bereavement services of the hospice team to cope with their tremendous loss.

Severe lung diseases like CF and COPD don't lend themselves readily to the typical 6-month prognosis required by most insurers for entering hospice care. For many patients, death occurs relatively unexpectedly during a flare-up of an otherwise gradual illness. The palliative care team can play a critical role by emphasizing the holistic aspects of care and providing options and information as the patient's needs change. Symptom management and patient comfort and autonomy remain the goals for palliative care. On those occasions when a prognosis has been established, hospice care can be offered as a continuation of the palliative process.

12 | **Patients with renal disease**

End-stage renal disease (ESRD) is the term used to describe a degree of chronic renal failure that, without dialysis or kidney transplantation, would end the patient's life. Many such patients have complex and special needs. Many are elderly. (See *Facts about end-stage renal disease.*) All ESRD patients need palliative care, careful efforts to maintain quality of life and, eventually, end-of-life care.

Currently, there's no cure for ESRD. The patient's options include only hemodialysis, peritoneal dialysis, kidney transplantation, or death. Clearly, ESRD patients and their families face many decisions about life-prolonging versus palliative therapies. Ideally, palliative care increases as curative care decreases, and it encompasses all aspects of illness through death and bereavement. (See *Models of end-of-life care.*)

Facts about end-stage renal disease

- Almost half of people with end-stage renal disease (ESRD) are older than age 65.
- More than 72,000 dialysis patients die each year.
- About 1 in 4 patients who die of ESRD do so because they withdrew from treatment.
- Most patients with ESRD also have other diseases that contribute to their deaths.
- Almost two-thirds of patients with ESRD die as hospital inpatients.
- Few patients with ESRD die in hospice care.

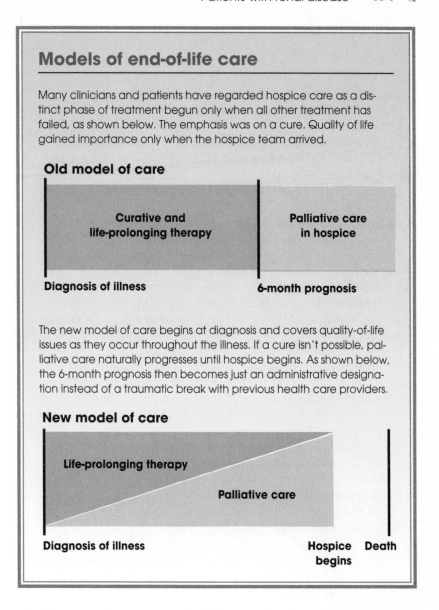

Models of end-of-life care

Many clinicians and patients have regarded hospice care as a distinct phase of treatment begun only when all other treatment has failed, as shown below. The emphasis was on a cure. Quality of life gained importance only when the hospice team arrived.

Old model of care

| Curative and life-prolonging therapy | Palliative care in hospice |

Diagnosis of illness **6-month prognosis**

The new model of care begins at diagnosis and covers quality-of-life issues as they occur throughout the illness. If a cure isn't possible, palliative care naturally progresses until hospice begins. As shown below, the 6-month prognosis then becomes just an administrative designation instead of a traumatic break with previous health care providers.

New model of care

Life-prolonging therapy

Palliative care

Diagnosis of illness   **Hospice begins**   **Death**

When caring for a patient with ESRD, as with other terminal illnesses, you'll need to address both physical and psychosocial issues for both patient and family. You'll play an essential role in assessing and managing the patient's symptoms, including pain. And you may have to help with such difficult decisions as when to stop dialysis.

Assessment

Normally, the kidneys serve many functions, including:
■ regulation of osmotic pressure through absorption or excretion of sodium chloride and water
■ regulation of fluid volume using antidiuretic hormone and water
■ regulation of electrolytes, such as sodium, potassium, calcium, phosphorus, and magnesium
■ regulation of pH through hydrogen ion excretion and sodium bicarbonate absorption
■ excretion of wastes, such as urea, creatinine, uric acid, and ammonia
■ secretion of hormones, such as erythropoietin and renin.

Damage to the kidney's functional unit—the nephron—can render it nonfunctional and reduce the kidneys' ability to carry out its normal duties. The glomerulus, a tuft of capillaries in the nephron, filters all blood entering the kidney. The glomerular filtration rate in a healthy adult averages about 120 ml/minute. If that figure falls to less than about 20% of normal, a series of events begins and may lead to chronic renal failure. (See *Course of chronic renal failure.*)

Symptoms of uremia most always occur if glomerular filtration rate (GFR) is less than 10% of normal. In fact, there's a direct relationship between a decreased GFR and metabolic changes that result from the kidneys' inability to regulate electrolytes, fluid, and acid-base balance and to excrete metabolic wastes and secrete hormones.

Several diagnostic measures are used to assess the presence of ESRD. These include a family history, blood tests, urine examination, kidney biopsy, and X-rays. The most common laboratory tests include:
■ blood urea nitrogen (BUN) level
■ serum creatinine level
■ BUN-to-creatinine ratio
■ creatinine clearance
■ biochemical profile, including the electrolytes sodium, potassium, magnesium, phosphorus, and calcium
■ complete blood count
■ urinalysis

As ESRD progresses, BUN and serum creatinine levels increase, urine creatinine clearance decreases, serum potassium level increases, phosphorus level increases, calcium level decreases, and hemoglobin level and hematocrit decrease. Lack of dialysis would result in these values remaining abnormal and would lead to death.

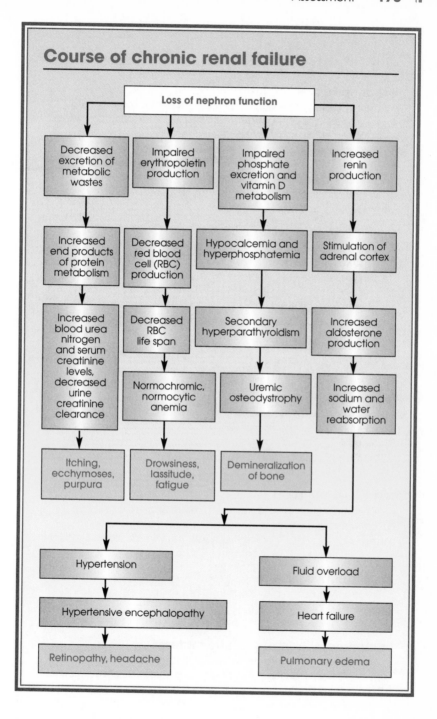

Course of chronic renal failure

Loss of nephron function

Decreased excretion of metabolic wastes → Increased end products of protein metabolism → Increased blood urea nitrogen and serum creatinine levels, decreased urine creatinine clearance → Itching, ecchymoses, purpura

Impaired erythropoietin production → Decreased red blood cell (RBC) production → Decreased RBC life span → Normochromic, normocytic anemia → Drowsiness, lassitude, fatigue

Impaired phosphate excretion and vitamin D metabolism → Hypocalcemia and hyperphosphatemia → Secondary hyperparathyroidism → Uremic osteodystrophy → Demineralization of bone

Increased renin production → Stimulation of adrenal cortex → Increased aldosterone production → Increased sodium and water reabsorption

Hypertension → Hypertensive encephalopathy → Retinopathy, headache

Fluid overload → Heart failure → Pulmonary edema

Effects of end-stage renal disease

Renal system
- Oliguria results from a decreased glomerular filtration rate (GFR).
- Hyperkalemia results from decreased GFR and metabolic acidosis.
- Metabolic acidosis results from the kidney's inability to excrete hydrogen ions and reabsorb sodium and bicarbonate.
- Hyperphosphatemia and hypocalcemia develop because the kidney can't excrete phosphorus.
- Hypotension and dehydration may occur during or after dialysis and may lead to further kidney ischemia.

Cardiovascular system
- Hypertension results or worsens from fluid overload, stimulation of the renin-angiotensin mechanism, or the absence of prostaglandins.
- Left ventricular hypertrophy, heart failure, or both may result from volume overload.
- Arrhythmias may result from hyperkalemia, hypermagnesemia, acidosis, and decreased coronary perfusion.

Respiratory system
- Pulmonary edema results from heart failure and fluid overload.
- Pleuritis may result from toxic byproducts of metabolism.

Gastrointestinal system
- Anorexia, hiccups, nausea, and vomiting occur with uremia.
- GI bleeding may result from coagulation abnormalities and uremic gastric irritation.
- Peptic ulcer disease and symptomatic diverticular disease are common in chronic renal failure.

Neurologic system
- Peripheral neuropathy leads to burning feet or restless legs.
- Seizures, forgetfulness, a shortened attention span, impaired reasoning and judgment, and central nervous system depression may result from circulating toxic substances.

Reproductive system
- Erectile dysfunction may result from physiologic and psychosocial causes.
- Libido may decrease from physiologic and psychosocial changes.

Immune and hematopoietic systems
- Anemia may stem from decreased erythropoietin production, glomerular filtration of erythrocytes, or bleeding from platelet dysfunction.
- Malaise, weakness, and fatigue are very common.
- Platelet dysfunction may accompany uremia.
- Infection and sepsis commonly occur from decreased immunity.

ESRD adversely affects most body systems. (See *Effects of end-stage renal disease.*) When implementing end-of-life care, carefully assess for these effects and plan your care to increase the patient's comfort.

Treatment

Life-sustaining treatment for ESRD includes hemodialysis, peritoneal dialysis, or renal transplantation. Drug therapy and diet management also play a vital role in treating ESRD.

Hemodialysis

In hemodialysis, blood is removed from the patient, filtered through an external artificial kidney, and returned to the patient. In an emergency, blood may be drawn from a central venous catheter. For long-term use, blood may be drawn through an arteriovenous (AV) fistula or AV graft. (See *Access devices for hemodialysis*, page 176.)

 ALERT Don't measure the patient's blood pressure or perform a venipuncture, except for dialysis, in the limb with the access device. Check the device regularly for a bruit and a thrill. Loss of a bruit may indicate occlusion of the access site.

The hemodialysis process involves cleansing the blood of toxic wastes such as urea and creatinine, restoring electrolyte balance, eliminating extra fluid from the body, and returning the cleansed blood to the patient through the access site. A major component of this process is dialysate, a solution of glucose and salts, which facilitates the process. At no time during dialysis do dialysate and blood mix. This entire process takes about 3 to 5 hours. Typically, patients are dialyzed three times a week.

A patient who needs hemodialysis will have periodic blood tests. He'll also be weighed before and after each dialysis session. Both the laboratory work and body weight help determine the efficacy of treatments and how well the patient is adhering to the therapeutic regimen.

Risks of hemodialysis include:
- acute anaphylactic reaction during dialysis
- acute hemolysis of red blood cells during dialysis
- air embolism before, during, or after dialysis
- arrhythmias
- dialysis disequilibrium syndrome (nausea, vomiting, headache, confusion)
- hypotension (15% to 30% of patients)

Access devices for hemodialysis

A double-lumen, cuffed hemodialysis catheter is used in acute hemo-dialysis. The red adapter is attached to the line through which blood is pumped from the patient. After blood passes through the dialyzer, it returns to the patient through the blue adapter.

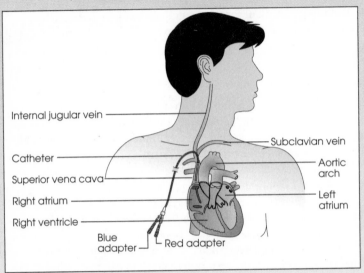

An internal arteriovenous fistula is created by a side-to-side anastomosis of the artery and vein. A graft can also be established between the artery and vein.

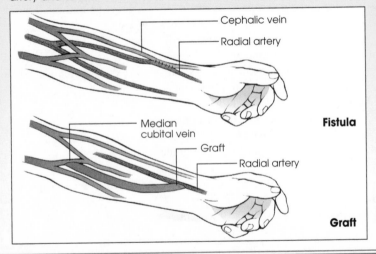

- inadequate filtering of waste products, indicating hemodialysis inadequacy
- infection, especially with central catheters
- muscle cramps
- thrombus formation in the blood access device.

Peritoneal dialysis

In peritoneal dialysis, dialysate is infused into the peritoneal cavity, and blood is cleansed across the vascular wall of the cavity. The vascularity of the peritoneal cavity along with the dialysate facilitates waste removal, electrolyte regulation, and fluid removal.

Three types of peritoneal dialysis are currently being used: continuous ambulatory peritoneal dialysis, continuous cycler-assisted peritoneal dialysis, and nocturnal intermittent peritoneal dialysis, of which continuous ambulatory peritoneal dialysis is the most common. (See *Continuous ambulatory peritoneal dialysis*, pages 178 and 179.) The patient may feel mild back pain or abdominal fullness during the procedure.

The most common risks of peritoneal dialysis are peritonitis and infection of the skin around the Tenckhoff catheter. The procedure also can lead to problems with glucose metabolism because of the concentration of glucose in the dialysate.

Diet and drug regimens

Diet management in ESRD reflects the patient's clinical condition and involves special attention to protein, salt, potassium, phosphorus, and calcium intake. Another major dietary consideration is the amount of fluid consumed each day. Fluid restriction is also based on the patient's clinical status.

Vitamin and mineral supplements are a routine part of management for patients with ESRD. Other drugs most often routinely included in the treatment regimen are those needed to treat hypertension and those needed to treat hyperkalemia, hyperphosphatemia, and hypocalcemia.

Hyperkalemia is the most common cause of sudden death in the ESRD patient. Usually, it's related to dietary indiscretions, missed dialysis, or missed drugs. For some patients, the complexity of the illness and the intensity of management it requires to sustain life simply become too burdensome.

Continuous ambulatory peritoneal dialysis

Continuous ambulatory peritoneal dialysis is a useful alternative to hemodialysis in patients with renal failure. Using the peritoneum as a dialysis membrane, it allows almost uninterrupted exchange of dialysis solution.

In this procedure, a Tenckhoff catheter is surgically implanted in the abdomen, just below the umbilicus. A bag of dialysis solution is attached to the tube using sterile technique, and the fluid is allowed to flow into the peritoneal cavity, as shown. This takes about 10 minutes.

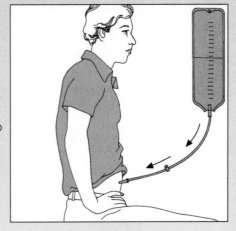

The dialyzing fluid stays in the peritoneal cavity for several hours. The approximate dwell-time for daytime exchanges is 5 hours; for overnight exchanges, the dwell-time is 8 to 10 hours. During the day, the bag may be rolled up and placed under a shirt or blouse, as shown, and the patient can go about normal activities while dialysis takes place.

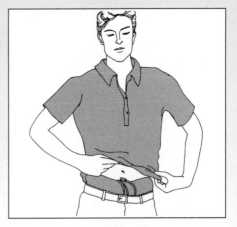

(continued)

Continuous ambulatory peritoneal dialysis *(continued)*

After each dwell-time, the patient drains the dialysis solution from the peritoneal cavity via gravity flow by unrolling the bag and suspending it below the pelvis, as shown. Drainage takes about 20 minutes.

After the fluid drains, the patient uses sterile technique to connect a new bag of dialysis solution and fills the peritoneal cavity again. Four to six exchanges of fresh dialysis solution are infused each day.

This form of dialysis offers the unique advantages of a simple, easily taught procedure and patient independence from a special treatment center.

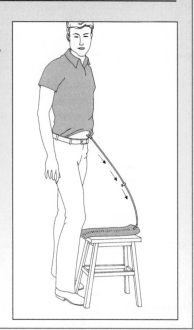

End-of-life care

ESRD may cause symptoms in virtually every body system. You'll need to address them diligently during end-of-life care. Pain is a priority problem for these patients, and you should anticipate the need for pain relief. There may be bone pain from decreased mineralization, abdominal pain from increased kidney size or fluid accumulation, or pain and muscle spasms from a decreased ability to eliminate toxins. Usually, opioids combined with acetaminophen should be used instead of those with aspirin or NSAIDS to decrease the risk of bleeding. Other problems, such as a metallic taste in the mouth, generalized edema, headaches, itching, and insomnia may require various treatments to alleviate symptoms.

Besides easing the patient's symptoms, you probably will need to help the patient and family through one of their most difficult transitions: deciding on and accomplishing the patient's withdrawal from dialysis.

Often, this topic arises when dialysis causes complications that diminish the patient's quality of life. Other reasons may include acute complications, such as dementia, stroke, and cancer. Some patients may prefer not to start dialysis at all. Here are some general principles to remember in preparation for this difficult transition:

■ The discussion should include the patient, family, and health care team.

■ Legal documents—such as advance directives and informed consent to treat or withdraw from treatment—are in place.

■ The patient knows the estimated prognosis for his condition.

■ Conflicts are resolved between patient, family members, and health care providers through effective communication.

■ The patient understands situations in which withholding or withdrawing from dialysis is appropriate.

■ Provision is made for time-limited trials of dialysis, if needed, while the patient considers his options.

■ Referrals are made to palliative care specialists if the patient chooses to withhold or withdraw treatment.

These principles emphasize the patient's right to honest, complete information with which he can make an informed decision. It's important that you and other health care providers establish a relationship with the patient that fosters his ability to discuss his wishes.

Roughly 1 in 4 patients with ESRD chooses to stop dialysis, and most of those who do die within a few days or weeks of stopping. These patients can anticipate having a variety of symptoms, including:

■ moderate to severe lethargy and malaise

■ Kussmaul's respirations, including periods of tachypnea and periods of apnea

■ auditory and visual hallucinations

■ agitation

■ anorexia, decreased fluid intake, and then dysphagia

■ chills and fever

■ constipation or diarrhea

■ discolored urine, if the patient is producing urine

■ muscle twitching or myoclonus

■ pain.

Ensuring the quality of end-of-life care takes an experienced interdisciplinary team working together with the patient and family. (See *Hospice referral: Human moments.*)

Remember that some elements of end-of-life care are fixed and some are modifiable. For example, the disease is fixed, as is the prognosis. The patient's life's experiences, psychosocial background, and cultural heritage also are fixed. Modifiable elements include pain, fatigue, drowsiness, in-

EXPERT INSIGHTS

Hospice referral: Human moments

Last week a physician wrote an order directing "social services to dis-
cuss hospice with patient." Nothing in the progress notes indicated
that the physician had discussed the patient's prognosis with her. I felt
uncomfortable with this request, so I phoned the physician. He didn't
take my call, but his receptionist said, "The doctor wants you to ar-
range for inpatient hospice because the family can't take care of the
patient any more."

I don't feel qualified to have this kind of discussion with a patient I
barely know. Should this be my responsibility? — C.P., Va.

Discussing hospice care entails discussing the prognosis. That's the
physician's job, not yours. The patient may have questions about
treatment options that you can't answer. Check your job description
and the policies and procedures for case managers. Ask your nurse
manager to intervene if needed.

Arranging for palliative and hospice care requires a dialogue that
no one really wants to have, physicians included. But our patients and
their families deserve nothing less.

I was in a similar situation when a young physician, Dr. Hall, wrote
an order for me to talk with his patient, Jane Lee. He not only wanted
me to discuss hospice placement, but he also wanted me to inform
her that it wasn't cancer that was killing her, but heart failure.

Believing he was better qualified than I to discuss her medical condition, I declined to act as his surrogate but offered instead to accompany him to her bedside. I pulled a chair up to the bed for him. He
reached out and gently took Jane's hand. But when he told her that
she couldn't go home, she abruptly withdrew it. She was obviously
overwhelmed.

"I thought you said the cancer wasn't so bad right now," she said.

"Yes, well, no," Dr. Hall stammered. "What I meant was, it's your
bad heart that's the problem now. Your breathing has gotten much
worse even with the medication and increased oxygen."

She lay back and shut her eyes.

Dr. Hall started to get up, but I pressed my hand on his shoulder,
pushing him firmly into the chair. I spoke softly, "Jane, Dr. Hall cares
about you, and all of us feel terrible that we can't fix this. You may ask
either of us any questions about anything."

(continued)

Hospice referral: Human moments (continued)

I felt Dr. Hall tremble slightly, but I wanted him to realize that words are the most powerful tools a physician has. When such information is given poorly, his patients will never forgive him. But when bad news is given well, his patients will never forget him.

Finally, Jane opened her eyes and took Dr. Hall's hand. "I don't blame you, you know. I just hoped I'd have a little more time."

"I'm so sorry," he said.

I left the room. Dr. Hall, the physician, had invited Kevin Hall, the human, to his patient's bedside. What a fine team they made.

— JOY UFEMA, RN, MS

---

somnia, and other physical discomforts that can be reduced with proper palliative care. Some psychological and cognitive symptoms are also modifiable.

Respectful inquiry and data gathering is a must in identifying fixed elements and modifiable ones. The fixed elements are individual to the patient and can be acknowledged and discussed but not changed. The modifiable elements can and often should be changed through appropriate palliative care. Help the patient identify his expectations and needs, and help him set goals that are appropriate for available interventions. It isn't inevitable that the end-of-life process be unbearable for the patient. Many of the symptoms can and should be treated diligently.

Other modifiable elements that can be addressed in the plan of care are support systems and caregiving needs. ESRD affects not only the patient but the patient's social and support systems and caregivers. It's important that you know when to call on other members of the interdisciplinary team to facilitate work with families and caregivers. Keep in mind that certain health care workers specialize in working with children and their siblings and parents. These specialists can help you identify a child's fears and his understanding of illness, dying, and death.

Care of a dying child | 13

Like adults, children are eligible for all types of hospice care: routine, inpatient, continuous, and respite. Almost always, children receive hospice care at home or as inpatients.

However, a hospice can't bill for services if a patient is still undergoing aggressive treatment, and most parents want to continue treatment if their child's life has any chance of being spared. Consequently, most children who could benefit from hospice care never receive it, and few hospice programs focus specifically on children. Although most adult hospice programs will accept pediatric patients, most of the staff would be the first to admit that they're ill prepared to serve the needs of dying children. In fact, many hospice nurses choose to work only with adults, finding work with children too painful.

Two common reasons for children to need end-of-life care are end-stage cancer and grave congenital defects or birth injuries. Many other problems can bring a dying child to end-of-life care as well, including accidents, violence, genetic diseases, and almost every imaginable complication of illness or surgery. Families of dying children often are faced with the same painful decisions that families of dying adults must face, including withdrawing life support. (See *Letting Lisa go*, pages 184 and 185.)

Child care

If you're helping to care for a dying child, much of what you provide will mirror the types of care an adult would receive. In addition, keep these spe-

EXPERT INSIGHTS

Letting Lisa go

I'm caring for Lisa, age 10, who has a rare and aggressive brain tumor with a poor prognosis. Bright and articulate, she told me months ago that she wasn't afraid to die and didn't want to undergo chemotherapy. But her parents convinced her to give it a try, even though the response rate was less than 5%.

The treatment wasn't effective, and now Lisa is nearing the end of her life. She seems to have accepted this, but her parents won't give up. Yesterday I heard her dad say, "You can't die now; we need you!"

I'm deeply troubled by this and want to help the child, but how? — K.S., Ontario

This situation is extremely difficult for all involved, especially Lisa. She has to face dying and death without her family's support — because although they're physically present, they're not emotionally or spiritually available.

For Lisa's sake, her parents need to let her go. And you can be the catalyst that helps them take this step.

Sit privately with Lisa and ask if she feels like sharing what she's going through and how she feels about this cancer. If she does, ask her if she wants you to relay those words to her family or if she'd prefer to tell them herself. If she chooses the latter, ask if she'd like you to be present as her helper.

With your support, she may find the courage to speak to her parents

cial points in mind. (See *Guidelines for care of dying children and their parents*, page 186.)

Safe haven

As much as possible, keep the child's bed a safe haven. Try not to perform painful procedures while the child is in bed. Nurses who work in children's hospitals or designated pediatric units usually have policies to guide their practice and a designated procedure room to avoid the need to cause a child pain while in bed.

If you don't have the luxury of a procedure room and the patient is ambulatory or up in a wheelchair, consider going into another room. For example, you might be able to set up a sterile field on the kitchen table to perform I.V. or port maintenance.

about her wishes. She's probably tried to talk with them in the past but been discouraged by their distress.

In your role as Lisa's advocate, you might call her parents to her bedside and say something like this: "Lisa loves you so much and appreciates all you've done during these weeks and months. Now she has something very important that she needs to say."

Listening to their child say that she doesn't want to go on will be heartbreaking for Lisa's parents. But they need to hear the truth.

During the conversation, you might ask Lisa if she'd like to discuss her funeral or tell her family how she wants to be remembered. This is the time to identify her favorite music, readings, and people she'd like to have speak about who she was and why she was a great kid. You could suggest the idea of making a casting of her hand that she can give to her parents and grandparents. Or she might want to produce a short video as a personal way to say good-bye to friends and family.

Finally, I recommend that you talk about getting hospice involved. Lisa's parents may need help to honor her wish to avoid "heroic" interventions as death approaches. Hospice personnel can provide good counsel and support in this matter. They'll also provide bereavement follow-up for a year after Lisa dies, when her parents need compassion and emotional support as they adjust to life without their child.

— JOY UFEMA, RN, MS

To respect the child's privacy in the home, many procedures — such as urinary catheter or wound care — may have to be done in the child's room or even in the bed. And a patient who is immobilized and dying shouldn't be removed from bed regardless of age.

No lying

Never lie to a child, especially a child who is your patient. If a procedure is going to hurt, tell the truth. A patient who is dying needs to be able to trust you; if you lie, that bond of trust will not be possible.

Also, remember that the child is your patient first. Listen to what the child is saying, and respond according to the developmental level of the child, using words or actions he understands. Prepare the child ahead of time for any changes in the routine or new procedures. Be the child's advo-

---

Guidelines for care of dying children and their parents

- Never lie to the child.
- Keep the child's bed a safe haven whenever possible.
- Be the child's advocate first.
- Be careful what you say and how you say it.
- Consult with social services and spiritual providers to help parents let go of the child's life.
- Provide privacy to say good-bye after the death.
- Provide private access to a telephone.
- Help with transportation and food as needed, if the parents and child aren't at home.
- Refer the family to bereavement services, particularly those designed for parents.

---

cate, and help him express his thoughts and wishes to family and physicians if needed.

Family care

Each family of a dying child faces unique heartbreak. Family members won't always be rational, and they won't always be receptive to teaching and learning. Stress rarely brings out the best in people and, by default, you may be on the receiving end of the family's turbulent emotions at times. Stay calm and professional, and listen empathetically. Identify their most important need at the moment and work with them to meet it. They may be hungry, tired, financially stressed, or in need of time for their own personal hygiene or emotional outlets. They may also be struggling with emotional and spiritual distress, frustration, anger, denial, or grief. Helping the parents through this period can make them better able to be there for their child.

The sample cases included here offer an idea of the range of family issues that may arise when a child is dying. For clarity, each case tries to focus on one issue, even though many families have multiple issues. The patients and families are invented or composites; none represent real people.

Aban, a newborn

Baby Aban was the first child of a newlywed Muslim couple. Aban's mother was a teenager brought from the Middle East as the bride of the oldest son of an unassimilated Arab immigrant family who had been in the United States a few years. The young mother spoke only Arabic; her husband spoke limited English. Aban's father was only a few years older than his bride, with minimal education.

The couple lived with the groom's parents and his younger brothers and sisters. The groom's parents spoke only Arabic, and only Arabic was spoken in the home. The only members of the household who spoke English fluently were the younger children who had attended public school in the United States.

Silent arrival

Aban came into the world silently. His silence and floppy appearance alerted the hospital staff that he needed further evaluation. He was examined by the finest neonatal neurologists, and every possible test was done. The prognosis was grave. Aban had only brain stem function, which allowed him to breathe but little more. Despite having been told all of this in Arabic, neither of Aban's parents understood the severity and consequences of Aban's condition.

Aban appeared almost normal when he slept. However, when he was picked up, his deficits became apparent, and his sightless eyes spun wildly. Aban was floppy and doll-like and made no purposeful movement. Because he lacked reflexes and couldn't suck, he was fed through a nasogastric tube. Aban's parents were taught how to care for and tube feed their son, and they were given a hospice referral. Then baby Aban was sent home.

Parental denial

Baby Aban's case focuses on parental denial of the reality of a child's terminal state. (See *Aban, a newborn*.) Because Aban looked like a relatively normal newborn, his family had trouble understanding the severity of his condition. Perhaps they hoped there had been a mistake with the diagnosis and that the baby would improve.

Islam requires that extraordinary means be employed to prolong life, and Aban's father demanded that the infant be resuscitated when needed in the hospital. Aban's father learned cardiopulmonary resuscitation and resuscitated the infant several times after his discharge from the hospital.

Normally when a patient receiving hospice care is resuscitated or the family wants aggressive treatment, the hospice agency discharges the patient. In Aban's case, because of the language barrier and cultural issues, the hospice gave the family extra social work intervention and spiritual counseling and gave the family additional time.

Because the family didn't seem to comprehend the explanation of Aban's neurologic status or the results of sophisticated neurologic tests, a more basic approach was employed. The baby was given an additional neurologic exam in the home with his family present. During the test, the findings (and what the normal findings would have been) were translated into Arabic.

Aban didn't respond to light, sound, or other stimuli; he lacked even basic reflexes. Clearly, Aban wasn't simply weak or sick. He had no response. The Arabic translator explained that Aban's lack of higher brain function meant that he was blind, deaf, and unable to suck or voluntarily move his muscles. Each deficit was slowly enumerated in Arabic. Aban would never see or hear, never walk or talk, and never have any awareness.

Aban died shortly after his in-home neurologic exam; he was 27 days old. This time, his father didn't resuscitate him. Because no treatment could improve Aban's condition, allowing him to die when his heart stopped naturally was within Islamic law and could be perceived as being Allah's will. Social work continued to follow the family for bereavement support.

Nursing challenges

Bobby's situation reveals special care planning needs for children with developmental difficulties. (See *Bobby, a special-needs child.*)

A plan was devised to minimize the need to touch Bobby and to limit the number of people who visited the home. Although it required extra overtime and special commitment from his nurses, Bobby was visited almost exclusively by the three nurses he knew, 24 hours a day, seven days a week, until he died. Because he had an I.V. port, he was given a portable pump for continuous morphine infusion.

Bobby's grandmother moved into the home to help provide care, but Bobby's mother and grandmother were unwilling to attempt "medical things." They did agree to be trained in some tasks that would make Bobby's life less stressful.

For example, being touched by a nurse to remove the transparent dressing over his I.V. site wasn't working. Although the procedure wasn't painful, Bobby disliked the sensation and screamed continuously while the nurse removed the dressing. Oddly enough, Bobby tolerated the sterile procedure for the new transparent dressing fairly easily. To reduce Bobby's stress, his grandmother was taught how to remove the old transparent dressing. Although he still disliked the sensation, he could tolerate it without screaming when his grandmother removed the dressing.

The nursing visits were streamlined and conducted with the speed and precision of a pit crew at the racetrack. Bobby was told on the nurse's ar-

> ## Bobby, a special-needs child
>
> At age 7, the third child and only son of a divorced mother, Bobby had already experienced a lifetime of tragedy. Bobby's father had abandoned his family before his son was born. Bobby's mother loved her children desperately but had trouble supporting them.
>
> As a charming, loving toddler, Bobby had been struck by a car and suffered severe brain trauma. His sweet, cooperative disposition was replaced by a sullen, solitary nature. Bobby avoided physical contact and would pull away violently, shrieking when touched. He wasn't toilet trained and would tolerate only his mother or maternal grandmother as caregivers.
>
> ### Screams, shrieks, and tantrums
>
> Bobby rarely spoke, and his utterances were usually limited to one or two words punctuated by screams, shrieks, and tantrums. Often, his family could interpret his several degrees of screaming and shrieking. His response to stress and strangers was to scream. His response to pain and fear was to scream louder. His response to greater pain and fear was to scream even louder and become violent.
>
> Bobby was diagnosed with cancer at age 4. His mother requested that everything be done to prolong her son's life. Cancer treatment was difficult for Bobby, his family, and the staff, but his oncologist tried every available treatment without success.
>
> Now, at age 7, Bobby had reached the final stages of his terminal illness. His cancer was painful, and he needed continuous medication. However, Bobby was no more agreeable to being touched or visited by strangers just because he needed their help. Each nursing visit was an ordeal for both Bobby and the nurse, but admitting him to the hospital — requiring him to leave his home — was too stressful for Bobby to handle.

rival if the visit was "for him" or for his morphine pump. Bobby much preferred that the pump receive the visit because it meant that he wouldn't have to be touched.

Bobby was fairly cooperative with having a stethoscope touch his chest or having a thermometer under his arm because that didn't require the nurse to touch him. He was far less cooperative about having his blood pressure checked as he disliked the sensation of the cuff; consequently, blood pressure was rarely taken. When he had to be touched, an effort was made to touch him only with one hand and to touch only one area at a time. This approach was easier for Bobby to tolerate.

Caring for Bobby wasn't easy; the screaming and shrieking was nerve wracking for the nurses despite assurances from his mother that the pitch

Cindy, a pre-teen

Playing Frisbee on an unusually warm spring day, 12-year-old Cindy stepped into the street — and into the path of an oncoming car. Cindy suffered massive trauma to her brain and spinal cord. A magnetic resonance imaging scan served only to confirm everyone's worst fears. If she managed to survive the trauma to her brain, Cindy would be quadriplegic and ventilator dependent. Her brain was just beginning to swell, and the extent of Cindy's brain injury wouldn't be apparent for days. Her chance of even surviving those days was very small.

Cindy's parents listened to what the physician told them, unable to grasp the reality of the situation. Just hours before, their daughter was perfectly normal. Now they had absolutely no idea what to do. Everything medically possible was being done for their daughter, but there was little chance of her surviving.

The physician suggested that they call their family priest and speak with the hospice and palliative care nurse to ask questions and discuss options.

and volume of the vocalizations was his "normal" response to stress. In his way, Bobby did develop trust for his nurses; although the vocalizing was never completely absent, it wasn't continuous or as loud as it was initially. At the end, Bobby was comatose, no longer in pain or having to deal with stress by screaming. His mother, grandmother, and siblings were given bereavement support.

Sudden loss

Cindy's story reveals the difficulties of a sudden, accidental loss of a child's health. (See *Cindy, a pre-teen*.) This family had many questions. Fortunately, the hospice nurse who arrived to do the information visit had started her nursing career in the intensive care unit and could explain to Cindy's shell-shocked parents everything that was happening.

The parents were very confused. The one thing they remembered was that everything seemed to depend on how much and how fast Cindy's brain swelled. They wanted to know why that was so important and how a swollen brain could kill their daughter. Would that be painful?

There was no pressure to stop treatment or enroll in hospice, only answers to their questions and the assurance that hospice and palliative care would be available if they needed them. The nurse spoke briefly with the family priest, who said that he'd given the girl the sacrament of the sick (last rites) and would encourage the family to use the hospice bereavement support group if the child died.

Daniella, a teenager

Daniella had leukemia and, at 15, was tired and dying. Her divorced parents had spent years in legal proceedings against each other and, with each of Daniella's relapses, had escalated their legal battle, in part over their only child.

Daniella decided to move into her father's lakefront home for her final days, but being anywhere other than the neutral ground of the hospital was problematic for both her parents. Even as their daughter's death approached, Daniella's mother and father continued their bitter struggle, refusing to speak directly to each other. Only with heroic effort did the hospice social workers secure the most minimal compromises.

The family never had to make decisions about continuing aggressive treatment or stopping life support; Cindy's brain swelled quickly and massively, causing it to herniate. As the brain stem was forced downward, Cindy's heart stopped, and she died instantly and painlessly. Although their daughter had passed away, the parents knew her death had been painless and that bereavement support was available.

Family discord

In Daniella's case, her dying process was profoundly influenced by discord within the family. (See *Daniella, a teenager*.)

Daniella went home to die in her father's house. The hospice staff suggested using the family room as her sick room for many reasons. The ground floor family room had an outside entrance that allowed her mother to avoid her father. It also had a full bathroom and a lovely view of the lake. To avoid having to see or speak directly to each other, Daniella's parents hired a live-in nurse's aide. The aide was expensive, but her presence and an extra phone line installed in Daniella's room insulated the teenager from her parents' constant bickering.

Daniella's hospice nurse would speak with whichever parent was present and call the other on a cell phone. Anything to do with Daniella's drug therapy was explained in detail to both parents and written down.

Because of the lack of communication, all of Daniella's scheduled drug therapy was set up in advance by the hospice nurse. Because Daniella was 15 and still able to swallow pills, whichever parent was present could simply bring the dose when it was scheduled. To avoid accidentally overmedicating their daughter, the parent would then record the dose in a log book that the other parent could consult later.

The social workers tried to help the parents plan how they would deal with Daniella's decline and death. They outlined options for around-the-clock bedside care. They also asked the parents to work out who would be present when their daughter died; Daniella said she wanted both of them there. While they were still arguing about it, Daniella died suddenly in her sleep.

After a child's death

At any age, dying and death are emotionally charged. A child's death will affect parents in a uniquely personal way. How long it will take them to recover will be individual to them. Use language that will promote comfort and healing without guessing at the length of their period of grief. Encourage the family to use bereavement support if possible.

Be careful both in what you say and how you say it. Offer empathy by listening, but don't try to sympathize with them. Saying "I understand how you feel" isn't appropriate. Most bereaved parents won't feel comforted by it and may instead feel insulted.

Also, do your best to be tactful. Every word you say may be permanently etched into a parent's brain. For example, if a child dies in the hallway outside the recovery area after surgery, tell parents that their child died in recovery. If a child is brain dead after trauma, the parents may be asked about organ donation before the child is referred to hospice; advocate for the patient and family to make sure this process is pursued in the most humane, respectful way possible. If the parents wish to donate the child's organs, be supportive and make the appropriate referrals.

Parents of children who die in your care may need very specific things at the moment of their child's death and afterward. Immediately, they need privacy to say good-bye to their child. They also need access to a telephone to notify loved ones of the child's passing. When they're finished, they probably will be in no condition to drive and should be offered a ride home. Losing a child is a life-altering experience, not the time to be navigating multiple bus lines or subway transfers, particularly ones that involve counting change.

Don't assume anything about the family's financial condition. They may have been financially destroyed attempting to save their child's life. They may not even have enough money for funeral expenses. If the mother rushed to the hospital unexpectedly without her purse, she may not have pocket change to buy something from a vending machine.

Regardless of how much time families have to prepare for the death of a child, it is aberrant. It's a commonly held belief that parents aren't supposed to bury their children; children are supposed to grow up and eventually bury their parents. It's difficult for parents to let go of a child, even if the child is enduring great physical suffering. Virtually all families of dying children need extended bereavement support.

Guilt is especially problematic for families of dying children, regardless of the terminal diagnosis. However, when trauma or violence are the cause, the family may be especially angry, guilt-ridden, or both. The families of children who die suddenly and unexpectedly from trauma or violence may have particularly complicated grief issues.

Multiple deaths

The death of one child is devastating, but sometimes a house fire, a motor vehicle collision, or some other type of accident kills or critically injures multiple children or family members. The stress and emotional toll on living family members is unimaginable. Their needs are many, and they'll require multiple services and extensive follow-up support. Traumatic stress complicates the grieving process greatly.

Depending on the nature of the tragedy, hospice may not be contacted until after family members have already died, or there may be critically injured family members fighting for their lives and other family members who are dead. Realistically, surviving family members will be in a state of shock and disbelief. An entire family or all of their children may have died in a single event. If the family has clergy, contact them as the living or dead children are brought to the emergency department. If the family is unaffiliated, contact either a hospice or hospital chaplain to provide immediate support.

In this age of mass communication, the media may be clamoring to report the tragedy in detail. Advise the family to immediately appoint one person, friend, neighbor, or relative to be the spokesperson for the family to deflect some of the attention from grief-stricken parents. It's better to have a press conference and release a statement than to have the continued presence of people trying to get photos and quotes from family members.

Images of the accident scene may persist on the local news for months in cases of ongoing legal action or criminal activity, the images rebroadcast with each phase of the arraignment and trial of the person responsible for the fatality. It's devastating and detrimental to healing for grieving parents and others who knew the victims to see these images over and over.

Our first duty is to the grieving parents and the surviving family, but the grief process is going to extend to entire schools, clubs, and religious organizations with which the family was affiliated. Children have unique grief issues, but even children who barely knew the dead children may be profoundly affected by the deaths of a family of children from their school. Normally, the school district is notified and they will provide grief counseling to the entire school.

Survivors of the event may have highly complicated grief issues and possibly survivor guilt. They will struggle to find meaning in the tragedy. For some parents, organ donation may be both comforting and a means of having some part of their child live on. Families who avidly support organ donation will be very familiar with the program. Other families may be far less receptive to being asked about organ donation and may be deeply upset, even if state law requires that they be asked.

A surviving parent may literally need someone present 24 hours a day to remind them to eat, drink, take medication, sleep, and otherwise keep themselves going after such a loss. Parents may be suicidally depressed after losing their children regardless of having no responsibility for their deaths. A parent who feels responsible — because he lost control of the family car on a patch of ice, for example, or because she lit a kerosene heater that burned the family home — may be inconsolable.

Well-meaning friends and relatives will want to help but often don't know what to do. The presence of professionals can often provide some guidance for their efforts: bringing prepared food, doing chores for the family, donating money to assist with the funeral costs.

The funeral may be even more difficult, and this is a time when funeral directors are invaluable. They will take care of many of the notifications, such as notifying the children's school district, any club or sport organizations the children participated in, the professional organizations the parents may belong to, and alerting the family as to what needs to be done.

No matter what brings a child to end-of-life care and what setting or program the child is in, the ideal approach is to integrate palliation into every phase of care, escalating to full palliation as the patient reaches the end of life. Because of the particularly complicated grief involved in the death of a child, end-of-life care should always include ongoing bereavement support for the family.

PART THREE

Helping the family

14 Family and caregiver care

End-of-life care is a process that involves not only the patient, but also the family and significant others. Commonly, the patient's loved ones provide most of the patient's care, an endeavor that can be emotionally and physically exhausting.

One of the most difficult moments in end-of-life care arrives when the prognosis and the finality of impending death must be disclosed to the patient and any family members whom he chooses to tell.

Before starting this discussion, carefully consider the role and requirements of confidentiality. In addition to causing emotional difficulties, discussion of the patient's diagnosis, prognosis, and care choices may pose multiple challenges to maintaining confidentiality. The obligation of confidentiality both prohibits health care team members from disclosing information about the patient's care and encourages them to make sure that only authorized persons have access to the patient's information.

Although occasionally a physician may feel a need to share information about a patient with an inquiring spouse when the patient can't give his consent, doing so usually is unwise. Unless the spouse is at risk of harm directly related to the diagnosis, it's the patient's obligation to inform his spouse rather than that of the physician or another member of the health care team.

Once the ethical and legal ramifications of discussing the patient's mortality are considered, the moment for disclosing the information must occur. (See *Starting the end-of-life conversation.*) Many patients don't remember the details of their diagnosis and prognosis but recall every moment of the conversation in which the disclosure occurred. The health care team's competence during this time is crucial to the patient's ability to maintain trust in the patient–caregiver relationship.

Starting the end-of-life conversation

When it's time to talk with a patient and his family about starting end-of-life care, find a private space in which everyone can sit comfortably. Make sure the participants have been selected by the patient. Also make sure you have all relevant information at hand. You may want to focus only on the diagnosis and treatment in one session, and reserve discussion of the prognosis and coping for a second follow-up session.

Find out how much the patient knows.
Determine how much the patient understands and how he feels about about his illness. Then tailor your presentation accordingly.

Find out how much the patient wants to know.
Some patients want to know every detail. Others, especially those who are stunned by a prognosis they weren't expecting, may be able to handle little more than the main concepts. You may find that you need to repeat information several times and to break information into smaller chunks than originally intended.

Share the information.
Stop after providing each chunk of information to assess the patient's and family's level of understanding. Encourage the patient and family to explain their understanding of the material back to you. Remember to translate medical terms into basic English; avoid falling into lecture mode.

Respond to the patient's feelings.
Particularly if the patient seems to be stunned or overwhelmed, ask how he's feeling. It's important to understand the patient's feelings so you can respond appropriately as part of the patient's support system.

Plan and follow through.
Develop a concrete plan based on the patient's concerns and medical issues. Discuss it with the patient and family on a step-by-step basis, and contract with the patient to implement the next step. Make sure the patient knows how to reach the appropriate member of the care team if an emergency arises before the next planned contact or clinic visit.

If the patient or family begins to weep during this conversation, stop the session and take a break. Stay with the patient. Make sure you have tissues available. Start the session again when the patient seems ready — even if that means waiting until another day. Be prepared to answer the same ques-

Caregiver roles

- Helping the patient understand palliative care goals, services, and the care plan
- Accessing palliative care, such as obtaining pain medication at the patient's request
- Advocating for the patient to receive optimal palliative care
- Supporting decisions made by a competent patient
- Making decisions for a patient no longer able do so himself in keeping with his previously expressed wishes, either verbally or by advance directive
- Helping the patient express his needs to the care team, as needed
- Providing food and fluids when the patient needs assistance
- Performing personal hygiene tasks for the patient, when needed
- Maintaining a comfortable environment for the patient
- Helping with financial matters, as needed
- Arranging for food and supplies to be provided
- Managing social visits for a patient who is fatigued
- Giving medications as instructed or when needed
- Supporting the patient spiritually and emotionally
- Participating actively in the bereavement process

tions several times. The first answer may have been too technical for the patient or family to understand, or they may simply be too emotionally distressed to hear it.

Often, the caregivers in end-of-life care are family members. About one-fourth of American families have assumed the care of an older family member or an adult child with disabilities. More than 7 million Americans are caregivers to older adults. More than half of caregivers are women.

The caregiver role is a stressful one, and the person who assumes such a role risks having her own physical, emotional, and spiritual needs go unnoticed as the patient's illness and impending death take center stage. The closer the patient is to the end of life, the more important the caregiver becomes. Caregivers are essential in accomplishing the goals of palliative end-of-life care — the opportunity to verbalize partings, reconciliation, and the provision of support. The informal caregiver who is helping with end-of-life care fulfills several roles. (See *Caregiver roles*.)

Demands on the caregiver

The demands on informal caregivers have increased in every setting: inpatient hospice centers, long-term care facilities, hospitals, and home settings. Informal caregivers at home, in addition to their daily household tasks, typically assume responsibility for the patient's medical care. Medical tasks such as giving analgesics and managing symptoms now are delegated to these caregivers. In fact, it may fall to a caregiver to not only give an analgesic but also to make decisions about dosages.

Caregivers may be expected to manage home I.V. therapy, epidural catheters, and patient-controlled analgesia pumps. They may feel fear and guilt that the analgesic could ultimately hasten the patient's death. As the patient approaches death, caregivers may feel increasing hesitation and anxiety about giving analgesics for fear that a particular dose may cause the patient's death. This anxiety is increased tenfold if the patient is requesting assistance with suicide.

It can be especially difficult when the caregiver is the patient's spouse. (See *Tips for caregiving spouses,* page 200.) Not only is the caregiver losing the loved one's companionship but also intimacy, familial stability, and possible wage-earning capacity. The caregiver may transition from being "superman" to being invisible to the patient as the patient withdraws mentally and emotionally from the living world.

Caring for a patient with dementia causes a higher level of stress than caring for a patient with functional impairment from a different kind of chronic illness. A patient with Alzheimer's disease typically needs an average of about 70 hours of care weekly, with 62 of those hours usually provided by the primary caregiver. Keep in mind, however, that the degree of stress and burden perceived by the caregiver isn't correlated with the amount of time spent providing care. Active coping skills on the caregiver's part are linked with lower levels of caregiver stress.

Many agencies provide support and information to caregivers. (See *Caregiver resources,* page 302.) It's important that caregivers learn to recognize their own needs and develop strategies for meeting them. It may also help the caregiver and hospice team if the caregiver takes time to write down her perceived strengths and weaknesses as a caregiver. This can help the team develop a care plan that assists the caregiver where most needed.

COMFORT & CARE

Tips for caregiving spouses

Enlarge the family unit.
The exclusive relationship you've had with your spouse or partner may no longer be realistic because of the level of care your loved one now needs. If you try to handle everything yourself, you may be quickly depleted of energy, frustrated, and possibly depressed.

Communicate sensitively with your spouse.
If you try to be too stoic, your ill loved one may interpret you as lacking compassion. However, if you fully air all your feelings, you may disrupt the patient's equilibrium and allow the illness to control your relationship. Try to seek a workable balance between communicating your feelings and supporting your spouse.

Let yourself experience a full range of emotions.
Caregivers commonly become numbed by the demands of endless tasks and the challenges of strong emotions. Denying fear, guilt, and anger can lead to depression and may prevent you and the patient from feeling joy in your relationship.

Encourage independence.
If your loved one can no longer contribute to the family financially, urge him to stay involved with the financial decision making. The ill person must be allowed to exercise his remaining abilities to keep from being consumed by the sick role — creating an even greater burden for the caregiver.

Express empathy.
Validate the emotions of the ill person so he has permission to share his feelings.

Seek counseling.
Counseling can validate your experience, help you prioritize tasks, clarify when you should seek respite care, and decrease feelings of loneliness.

Depression

Caregiving doesn't cause depression, and not every caregiver develops depression. But the effort to meet all the patient's needs can lead a caregiver to sacrifice her own emotional needs to such an extent that even the most capable person would be stressed. The resulting feelings of anger, isolation, exhaustion, and guilt can exact a heavy toll from the caregiver.

Although depression has been the most frequently researched area of caregiver health, these people are also at high risk for development of anxiety. What's more, immune function tends to be lower, leading to a longer duration of viral illnesses. Caregivers tend to have a higher mortality risk as well. To assess for excessive caregiver burden, ask specific questions. (See *Assessing caregiver burnout*, page 202.)

Women caregivers tend to experience depression and burnout at a higher rate than men, possibly because they tend to do most of the caregiving. Also, male caregivers tend to cope with depression differently than women. Men may be more apt to "self-medicate" with alcohol or excessive work. Their depressive symptoms are more likely to be anger, irritability, and a sense of powerlessness. Although male caregivers tend to hire assistance with home care duties, they also tend to have fewer confidants and tend to have fewer positive activities outside the home. The assumption that depression is a sign of weakness can make it particularly difficult for men to seek help when needed.

If the patient has dementia, the risk of caregiver depression doubles. Dementia-related symptoms such as wandering, agitation, hoarding, and engaging in embarrassing behaviors make it more difficult for a caregiver to rest and to solicit help from others. Sleep deprivation also may raise the caregiver's risk of depression. The caregiver may feel the need to stay awake whenever the patient is awake or restless.

Assessment

A caregiver with symptoms of depression should meet with both a primary physician and a mental health professional. The primary physician should pursue a complete physical examination to rule out any underlying disease processes or prescribed drugs that could contribute to the symptoms. The physical examination should include laboratory tests as well as an interview for mental status to determine if speech, memory, or thought patterns have been affected.

Because the caregiving role is likely to be a lengthy one fraught with many challenges, it is strongly recommended that a relationship be forged with a mental health professional so that guidance can be provided

Assessing caregiver burnout

To help detect caregiver burnout, ask questions such as these.
■ Do you feel that you're currently under a lot of stress? Describe the parts of your day that are most stressful for you.
■ Have you been feeling down lately?
■ Have you been feeling anxious or irritable lately?
■ Do your family and friends visit often? Do they visit enough? Do they telephone often?
■ Will your friends and family members stay with your loved one so you can have some time for yourself?
■ Do you have any outside help?
■ Does your loved one have any symptoms that are hard for you to manage?
■ What do you do to relieve your feelings of stress and tension?

throughout the end-of-life process. Such a professional may be located by asking a minister or rabbi, obtaining a referral from a physician, or consulting the caregiver's employer's employee assistance program.

A free introductory meeting may be possible to make sure the selected health care professional can work with the caregiver's emotional needs and style of coping. Advise the caregiver to clarify the cost of treatment, how much insurance will pay, and how many scheduled sessions the caregiver may be expected to have with the therapist. Certain kinds of questions may be expected in a mental health examination to determine the presence of depressive symptoms. (See *Assessing depression.*)

Management

Once the results of the physical and mental examinations have been evaluated, a course of treatment for the depressive symptoms will be recommended. Primary treatment options include psychotherapy and antidepressant drugs. Antidepressants are particularly useful if the depression has progressed beyond the mild stage. They provide relief of symptoms over 4 to 6 weeks and can provide a higher quality of life when combined with ongoing psychotherapy.

A depressed caregiver may feel exhausted, helpless, and hopeless. (See *Caregiver burnout*, pages 204 and 205.) Negative thoughts and feelings may even cause the person to consider suicide if he doesn't realize they're part of the depression and not an accurate reflection of his existing situation. To help a caregiver cope with depression, make suggestions such as these.

Assessing depression

To help determine whether a caregiver is developing depression, ask questions such as these.

- Have you noticed any changes in how you're feeling, thinking, eating, and sleeping in the past 2 weeks?
- When did you first notice the symptoms? How long have you had them?
- How do they affect you? Are there things in your daily life that you can't or don't do anymore?
- Have you ever experienced these feelings before? If you have, did you receive treatment? What type?
- How often do you use alcohol or drugs (both prescription and non-prescription) each week? Do you use them to help you cope?
- Have you had any thoughts about death or suicide?
- Do you have any family members who have experienced depression? If so, did they receive treatment? What type did they receive?
- Besides assuming your role as caregiver for your dying loved one, have you experienced any serious loss, relationship difficulty, financial problems, or other recent changes in your life?
- Is there anything else you'd like to say to help me understand your situation more clearly?

- Set realistic goals when you're feeling symptoms of depression, and assume a reasonable amount of responsibility for tasks or problem-solving.
- Break large tasks into small ones. Set priorities, and concentrate only on essential tasks.
- Try to be around other people and to find someone to confide in.
- Determine which activities make you feel better, and do them. Examples might include getting light exercise, attending social or community events, attending religious functions, or seeing a movie or sports event.
- Realize that your mood will improve gradually, not immediately, even if you take a prescribed medication for depression.
- Postpone important decisions and life-changing transitions until your symptoms have lifted. Also, discuss these potential changes with people you trust, people who know you well and can give you a more objective view of your situation.
- Expect a gradual reduction in negative thinking as the depression responds to treatment.
- Let family and friends help you.
- Use positive self-talk.

EXPERT INSIGHTS

Caregiver burnout

I'm a home hospice nurse caring for a terminally ill woman whose daughter is the live-in caregiver. Until recently, I found the house tidy and the patient bathed and dressed in beautiful pajamas whenever I visited. But last week, the house looked dirty and the patient was unkempt. Even so, the patient smiled and said, "Isn't my daughter an angel? I don't know what I'd do without her." When I glanced at the daughter, she abruptly walked out of the bedroom.

I'm not sure how to handle this. What do you think? — A.M., N.J.

Sounds as if the daughter would like to walk away from this whole situation. She's exhausted and needs help. When families become caregivers, they become our patients too.

The family dynamics here are unclear. The patient may not fully recognize her daughter's feelings of frustration, but her comment "I don't know what I'd do without her" may indicate that she senses a problem. Or she could be attempting to manipulate her daughter through guilt: Surely an "angel" wouldn't abandon her mother?

Speak privately with the daughter, beginning (and ending) the conversation with something postive, such as, "You're doing a marvelous job of caring for your mom." Acknowledge how difficult her task is, and stress that no one can do it alone. Encourage her to share the frustrations and rewards of caring for her mother.

■ Attend classes and meetings available through caregiver support organizations to help you learn and then practice effective problem-solving and coping strategies for caregiving.

Many patients wish to die in the security and comfort of their own homes. This may cause some caregivers to feel that they have no choice but to assume the caretaking role. This pressure can be reduced by open discussion between the patient, informal caregiver, and the health care team. The discussion should include the possible need to return to institutional care before death.

Assure the patient and family that the palliative care team will be there to help the patient move from home to institutional care. Finally, make sure that home caregivers have a range of services available to help them and to reduce the risk of burnout and depression.

Then ask how she feels about expanding the caregiving team. This could mean adding another hospice volunteer, asking other family members to take a shift, or hiring a nurse or a sitter, depending on her mother's care needs.

Another option is respite care. For example, the daughter could get a 5-day breather if the patient is transferred to a nursing facility that provides these services. In such a facility, patients are treated according to the hospice philosophy of comfort care only. The hospice agency pays the respite provider, and Medicare pays the hospice agency.

If none of these options gives the daughter the relief she needs, you may need to suggest placing her mother in an inpatient hospice center or a nursing home. This will be a sensitive issue for both women. Like most of us, the patient probably would prefer to die at home among familiar surroundings, and her daughter probably feels obligated to make that possible.

Both of your "patients" would benefit greatly from a visit by the hospice social worker. Having an honest, open dialogue about their true feelings and fears is the first step toward finding a workable solution and repairing what may be a growing rift in their relationship. Their last days together shouldn't be tainted with resentment. They both deserve so much more.

— *JOY UFEMA, RN, MS*

Respite and stress relief

If a caregiver doesn't receive respite on a regular basis, the health care team should encourage her to request this assistance and also should help find such relief. Adult day-care services can be a source of respite and also can provide a creative outlet for a patient with cognitive change.

Also, list the caregiver's usual strategies for stress relief, and evaluate whether they're emotion-focused or problem-focused. Examples of emotion-focused strategies include worrying and self-accusation. Examples of problem-focused strategies, characteristic of caregivers with a lower degree of burnout, include confronting issues and seeking information.

Active coping strategies, such as viewing the larger picture beyond the illness, are linked with a lower risk of depression among caregivers as well.

Coping skills for caregivers

To help a caregiver cope, offer suggestions such as these.
■ Educate yourself about your loved one's disease and how it may affect his behavior, emotions, and physical function.
■ Find sources of help. These may include other family members, friends, churches or synagogues, your workplace, and the local Area Agency on Aging.
■ Protect your personal time, and make sure to do things you enjoy.
■ Make time to exercise, eat well, and sleep adequately.
■ Use your personal network of family and friends for support, or locate a support group for caregivers in your area.
■ Notice symptoms of depression in yourself, such as crying more than usual, sleeping more or less than usual, lack of interest in normal activities, and an increased or decreased appetite. If these symptoms persist, talk with your physician.
■ Consider how you'll feel when your role as caregiver ends; what will you do then?

The caregiver should be able to visualize a moment when her life will resume and she will no longer be a caregiver. Support groups may be extremely beneficial and may reduce a caregiver's feelings of loneliness or isolation. There are several suggestions that may increase a caregiver's coping skills. (See *Coping skills for caregivers.*)

Self-care

Family caregivers of any age are less likely than non-caregivers to practice preventive health care and self-care. The combination of loss, prolonged stress, the physical demands of caregiving, and the aging process all place the caregiver at high risk for significant health problems and untimely death.

Caregivers tend to experience sleep deprivation, poor eating habits, failure to exercise, failure to engage in self-care during illness, and postponement or elimination of their own medical appointments. One-third of caregivers describe their own health as fair to poor. Many worry that they won't outlive the person for whom they provide care.

For caregivers to take responsibility for their own physical health, they must identify the attitudes and beliefs that are blocking them. (See *Why caregivers neglect their health.*) Failing to perform self-care may be a lifelong pattern, with caring for others being an easier and more rewarding option.

Why caregivers neglect their health

Caregivers may neglect their own physical health for these common reasons.

■ They think they must prove themselves worthy of the patient's affection.

■ They think they're being selfish if they put their needs first.

■ They get frightened when they think of their own needs.

■ They have trouble asking for what they need and feel inadequate asking for help.

■ They feel responsible for the patient's health.

Because our actions result from our thoughts and beliefs, negative attitudes and false perceptions can make caregivers try to control what is uncontrollable—the patient and the disease process. This maintains a constant feeling of failure and frustration and furthers a tendency to ignore the caregiver's own needs. Once barriers to maintaining personal physical and emotional health have been identified, the tools for effective self-care can be collected. One major way to maintain personal physical health is by reducing stress. (See *Five factors in caregiver stress.*)

Five factors in caregiver stress

1. Whether the caregiving role was assumed voluntarily. A caregiver who feels pressured into assuming the role is more likely to feel resentment.

2. The caregiver's relationship with the patient. If the caregiver assumed the role in hopes of healing an emotional rift, and the healing fails to occur, the caregiver may feel regret and discouragement.

3. The caregiver's coping abilities. How the caregiver coped with stress in the past can predict how she'll cope with stress now. Current coping strengths should be identified and expanded.

4. The caregiving situation. Typically, caring for a person with dementia is more stressful than caring for someone with a physical disability.

5. Support from family and friends. The availability of support, and the caregiver's willingness to accept it, can help reduce the caregiver's level of stress.

A caregiver's physical health can be greatly improved by a willingness to accept offers of help from others. Many caregivers are reluctant to admit that they have trouble handling everything on their own. Urge them to accept help, even with small tasks such as collecting a short list of items from the local market or sitting with the patient while the caregiver walks around the block or the neighborhood.

Communication

Another tool to promote physical, mental, and emotional health in caregivers is constructive communication. When a caregiver can communicate in ways that are clear, assertive, and constructive, she's much more likely to be heard and to receive the support she needs. Provide a few basic guidelines to help promote constructive communication. (See *Four principles of constructive communication.*)

Another crucial avenue of communication is with the physician. Along with performing household chores, shopping, and providing transportation and personal care, about 40% of caregivers also give drugs, injections, and medical treatments. Most of these caregivers say they need ready access to professional advice about these drugs and treatments. And although these caregivers usually will discuss the patient's needs openly with the physician, rarely will they discuss their own health.

When possible, urge the caregiver to make an appointment with the physician to discuss her own health needs in addition to the patient's. Suggest that she make a list of concerns and problems before the visit. Urge her to discuss any changes in the patient's symptoms, drug therapy, or general health along with her own comfort and needs in the caregiving situation.

The caregiver should make certain that the office staff understands her need for a particular appointment time if that's the case. If waiting time needs to be reduced or multiple questions asked, the first or last appointment of the day might be best. The office staff should be reminded of the caregiver's special needs upon arrival to the appointment. If the caregiver has trouble remembering details or needs to talk about multiple topics, urge her to bring someone with her to help remember the physician's advice or to ask the physician about the possibility of tape-recording or writing down important points of the discussion.

Also, keep in mind that many caregivers feel more comfortable asking questions of a nurse rather than a physician. You can serve as a valued resource for information such as preparation for surgical procedures, various laboratory tests, and home management of drug therapy.

Four principles of constructive communication

1. Use "I" messages rather than "you" messages. This allows feelings to be expressed without placing blame or causing others to become defensive.
2. Respect the rights and feelings of others. This recognizes the other person's right to express feelings without intentionally causing hurt.
3. Be clear and specific. Speak directly to the person; this shows respect for the other person's opinion. When both parties speak directly, the likelihood of reaching a clear understanding increases.
4. Be a good listener. This is the most important aspect of the communication process.

Spiritual and financial health

Spiritual health

Another core need for caregivers is spiritual health — however the particular person defines it. Religious practice helps maintain physical health. Regular churchgoers live longer; have a lower risk of dying from diseases such as arteriosclerosis, emphysema, cirrhosis, and suicide; and recover more rapidly when illness does occur. These people also tend to have lower diastolic blood pressures and more stable mental health.

Spiritual care for the caregiver can be extremely important since the caregiver faced with the need to cope with illness, emotional trauma, and discouragement is vulnerable and may feel desperate. The next progression is the neglect of the physical body as the caregiver begins to suffer intensely from isolation, inability to attend church services or other spiritual activities outside the home, and the helplessness caused by the need to fill a multitude of roles that she's ill-prepared to assume.

Financial health

Every area of the caregiver's life — physical, emotional, and spiritual — can be stressed by the financial burden of assuming the caregiving role. On average, 40% of caregivers are also raising dependent children and 64% work at least part-time. A study by the Metropolitan Life Insurance Company estimated that caregivers on average lose more than $650,000 in reduced salary and retirement benefits during the course of providing care.

Most caregivers have to create and follow a household budget to keep from threatening their own future. If the family member receiving care owns his own home, he may consider a reverse mortgage to help pay for the cost of receiving care. It allows a homeowner age 62 or older to borrow against the equity in her home as a line of credit, a lump sum, or monthly payments. The homeowner does not need to repay a reverse mortgage as long as he lives in the home. The loan is repaid when the owner sells the home or dies. The estate can repay the reverse mortgage with proceeds from the sale of the home or from another source of funds.

Another financial option is the purchase of an immediate annuity. This will prevent the scenario of an older person outliving his savings and requiring the caregiver to supplement this income. An annuity can be purchased from an insurance company for a lump sum and can guarantee a regular monthly payment for the remainder of the purchaser's life.

Expenses may be reduced for the caregiver of an older adult by researching governmental benefit plans or private and state prescription drug discount plans to reduce drug costs. Medicare recipients are eligible to purchase a private prescription drug discount card. Starting in 2006, Medicare added a prescription drug benefit to help seniors pay for drugs. Private insurers offer "medigap" plans for medical costs not covered by Medicare. Senior citizens with very low incomes may be eligible for Medicaid coverage along with Medicare. These "dually eligible" patients may be able to receive drug coverage through Medicaid. Some recipients also may be able to have their Medicare premiums, deductibles, and copayments paid by Medicaid.

Finally, investigate pharmaceutical companies that provide free drugs to low-income patients. Ultimately, the caregiver should discuss with family members the financial impact of assuming this role. They should be made aware of the various costs involved in providing care to the recipient. Consider setting up an Individual Retirement Account to replace retirement savings lost from the caregiver's employer. Also consider asking family members to pay the caregiver as an independent contractor for the care provided. This will allow the caregiver to set up a small-business type pension plan. The end result will be peace of mind for the caregiver, thereby ensuring a more therapeutic provision of care for the patient.

Support systems 15

When time and preparation allow, perhaps the most potent source of support for dying patients and their families is the hospice system, which provides multidimensional support services during the dying process and after the patient's death. Hospices nationwide are mandated to provide physical, emotional, spiritual, and bereavement support to patients, caregivers (whether relatives or paid staff), and families. These services can be provided to patients in their own homes, in assisted living facilities, in skilled nursing facilities, in hospice houses, and in hospitals.

The backbone of hospice care has always been to provide supportive care in the familiarity and comfort of the patient's own home surrounded by family, friends, and pets. If that's not possible, and if the patient doesn't meet the criteria required for inpatient hospice care (a short-term need for acute medical management of symptoms), then the palliative care team, the patient, and the family must discuss other available locations for care. Respite care (up to 5 inpatient days) or continuous nursing care (a short-term need for 8 or more hours of personal care in the home per day) may be available to support the primary home caregiver. A recent survey found that about half of hospice patients died at home, about one-fourth in a nursing facility, and less than 10% each in a hospice unit or hospital.

Home support

If the patient chooses to be cared for at home and already has caregivers, help them construct a list of equipment that may be needed. Focus on their abilities and needs. Ask the patient and caregivers what they think they might need. Don't force them to accept care items they prefer not to use. Arrange for the equipment to be delivered, preferably so that it will be there when the patient gets home. This intervention at the very first interview already provides emotional support to the patient and family.

Providing resources

In hospice care, a few things aren't negotiable, the main one being a minimum of one nurse visit every 14 days. Not many families opt for this minimal level of interaction, but there are some very private people who feel they can manage on their own. They may want help with drugs and answers to any questions that arise, but they also may want as few interruptions as possible. The acknowledgment of and respect for their needs is yet another form of silent support.

Depending on the hospice organization and the patient's choice, the patient will either retain his current physician or come under the care of a hospice medical director. Some attending physicians want to stay involved but prefer that a hospice physician with expertise in pain and symptom management take over that aspect of care. It's your responsibility to make sure the physician of choice knows of any changes in the patient's condition. This is especially important once the patient can no longer get to office visits. Occasionally, the patient's physician may choose to make home visits; however, this is a luxury for most physicians, so they rely on the hospice staff for information.

Regulations may state that an RN or case manager must see a patient within 24 hours of admission to hospice. Although most families are agreeable, some feel that their condition doesn't warrant an immediate visit or they're exhausted from weeks of treatments and travel to hospitals and really don't want another visit the day after admission to hospice. Remind them of the agency's availability 24 hours a day by telephone for questions, concerns, or problems. Make sure to document that the family has declined the visit and why and when you plan to see them.

Helping the caregiver

Often a family caregiver is also elderly or ill. In such cases, the hospice and palliative care team must monitor the health and abilities of the caregiver as well. Providing a volunteer so the caregiver can see her doctor, convincing the patient to accept a hospital bed or bedside commode to relieve physical demands on the caregiver, and teaching multiple family members to care for a patient can help maintain the health of the primary caregiver. It also helps to let them know how valuable their service and support is.

When you go out to see the patient and caregiver, assess their home and their specific needs once they are settled in. Perhaps additional equipment will be beneficial. Also, set up a home health aide schedule as needed. The home health aide may visit only two or three times a week to start. If more frequent personal care is needed or requested, the schedule will be adapted. Although the aide is in the home for personal care of the patient, she can also:

- provide respite for the caregiver to leave or have a nap or some quiet time
- provide a meal for the patient
- do the patient's laundry
- change the bed linens
- tidy the living area.

As well as performing these physical tasks, the aide develops a rapport with the patient and family and provides emotional and possibly spiritual support.

In hospice care, volunteers are another important part of the interdisciplinary team and provide support to patients and caregivers. Some of the services they may provide include:

- sitting with a patient while a caregiver goes shopping or to an appointment
- running errands for the family
- making support phone calls.

Some of the relationships formed between caregivers and volunteers continue for years. After the patient's death, the primary role of volunteers is weekly or monthly phone contact with the surviving family members.

As the patient begins to decline, you and the home health aide should instruct and model for the caregiver how to turn the patient in bed, help him transfer to a chair, change his bed, and provide mouth care. The staff should assess and evaluate the caregiver's abilities and needs and make recommendations with each contact.

Evaluate the patient's pain and comfort level each time you visit. Teach the caregiver how to evaluate them as well, so the caregiver feels better able to help the patient with drug therapy and other comfort measures. Teach the patient and caregiver about each drug in the plan of care, its actions, proper usage, and common side effects. Also explain other treatments as needed, such as oxygen therapy, urinary catheter care, and prophylactic skin care. As patients and caregivers gain new skills, their confidence will increase and they'll feel more empowered as part of the interdisciplinary team.

Complementary therapies

Complementary therapies such as massage therapy; physical, occupational, and speech therapy; and pet therapy may improve the quality of life for patients and caregivers. Other complementary therapies may be helpful as well. (See *Complementary therapies and hospice*.)

Massage therapy

Increasing numbers of hospices are including massage therapy as an integral part of patient and family care. Most patients who receive massage report reduced pain and anxiety and an improved sense of peacefulness. These are important indicators if we want to provide optimal physical and emotional support.

Physical, occupational, speech therapies

Physical, occupational, and speech therapy may have a role in supporting some terminally ill patients. The usual role for physical and occupational

---

Complementary therapies and hospice

Many patients bring their own experiences with complementary therapies with them into end-of-life care. They may feel strongly that a particular therapy has prolonged their life or increased their comfort. Support the patient's choices, and try to include the provider of complementary care in the interdisciplinary team. At times, techniques such as those listed here may be introduced to new patients who are struggling for comfort and not responding well to traditional therapies.

- Acupuncture
- Chiropractic
- Healing or Therapeutic Touch
- Herbal preparations
- Homeopathy
- Imagery
- Intercessory prayer
- Magnets
- Meditation
- Music therapy
- Qi gong
- Reflexology
- Reiki
- Shiatsu (acupressure)

therapy is to teach patients and caregivers how to use assistive equipment, transfer techniques, or adaptive techniques for activities of daily living. A speech therapist might work with a patient to improve swallowing, allowing him to drink or eat better and to better enjoy the taste and texture of foods. The speech therapist also might help a patient who's losing his speech to develop alternative communication methods.

Pet therapy

A popular complementary therapy, especially for institutionalized patients, is pet therapy. Bringing cats and dogs into a facility or even a private home can bring back memories and also the comfort of unconditional love that a pet can bring.

Financial support

Some hospice agencies have admission teams comprising both registered nurses and social workers. If a social worker hasn't been part of the initial visit, he should meet with the patient and family promptly after admission to review any financial questions and provide emotional support. The social worker can provide more detailed information on insurance, explain billing questions frequently encountered by caregivers, and help with a variety of family issues according to specific needs.

The social worker will spend time with the patient, family, and caregivers to listen to their concerns because each person may be in a different stage of the grieving process. Families with young children facing the death of a parent have different issues than those of a middle-aged child caring for an elderly parent. The social worker listens, teaches, facilitates, and models good communication skills.

If some family members are estranged, the social worker may help the patient resume contact if desired. Family dynamics may greatly impact the quality of care given in the home, and the social worker and all team members should work to alleviate discord and demonstrate good, safe care. (See *Family dynamics*, pages 216 and 217.)

EXPERT INSIGHTS

Family dynamics

I'm caring for a mentally retarded young woman who's dying of heart failure. Her elderly parents are legal guardians and have made appropriate medical decisions. The problem is her older sister, who's very argumentative. She constantly challenges the physician's orders and even her own parents' decisions on her sister's behalf. The parents seem stymied by her behavior, and the nurses feel defensive. Any suggestions? — H.M., Ontario

I can understand your frustration. I experienced a similar situation with a terminally ill patient, Kate, and her husband, Jon. A recovering drug addict, Jon spent countless hours at his wife's bedside, asking questions and raising issues with staff. Many of them found his behavior disruptive and his outlook unrealistic — especially his opposition to the do-not-resuscitate (DNR) order Kate's physician recommended. Perhaps influenced by his drug abuse history, they dismissed his often legitimate concerns.

After talking privately with Jon, I began to understand that his behavior with staff was an attempt to control a small but vitally important part of his life. I decided to help by empowering him. I began with the little things, saving the major decision about DNR status for later.

For instance, I might say, "Jon, I was thinking it might be refreshing to Kate if we shampooed her hair, but I wanted to run that by you first."

Or "Would it be okay with you if we turn Kate and put a pillow under that left leg?"

Spiritual support

One of the other members of the support team is the chaplain. When a patient starts end-of-life care, ask him and his family about their spiritual or religious preferences and whether or not they want to see a chaplain. It isn't unusual for a patient facing death to want to talk with a spiritual counselor even after being inactive in a religious institution for years.

Many chaplains are interdenominational, but a patient who belongs to a specific denomination or religion may wish to see a representative from his

He responded positively to those requests and began to act calmer. I decided it was time to sit with him again and discuss code status.

"Kate's very fortunate to have you as her advocate," I began. "You've been our go-to guy to help us make every decision that's in her best interest."

He smiled proudly. I touched his shoulder. "But I need to ask you to make the most important decision of all."

He interrupted me. "Yeah, I know. Her DNR."

"Yes, because if Kate..."

"Don't do it," he said. "She's had enough."

I gave him a big hug and then went to call Kate's physician.

You might consider a similar approach with your patient's sister. If her parents are elderly, she may have been the chief caregiver, babysitter, and "nurse" most of her sister's life. Now that role has been usurped by strangers.

Encourage her to be more, not less, involved in caregiving and decision making. Ask about her sister's favorite stuffed animals or blankets. Ask what position her sister finds most comfortable when she's lying down or sitting in a chair. Find out what kind of music her sister likes best. I think you'll see her behavior soften once you welcome her participation.

We all want to be valued and heard — especially when we're about to lose our most important job, a lifetime of caring for a loved one.

— JOY UFEMA, RN, MS

own faith. Local clergy generally are receptive to providing this service and understand the need for rapid response. Their role may be simply to bring a sacrament to the patient, but often they are called upon to give more in-depth support stemming from some lifelong spiritual questions.

Caregivers may have different spiritual beliefs and needs than the patient. Assess their individual needs and help them gain spiritual support as well. Caregivers may also have difficulty separating the patient's issues from their own. Provide private time with the staff or a spiritual support person so the caregiver can discuss conflicts, fears, or frustrations. Teach the caregiver ways to open up conversations with their loved ones and be supportive of the patient.

For various reasons, some patients wish to have a funeral but have no one to do the service. Chaplains will also step into this role and make all the arrangements along with a caregiver and family's input and also actually perform the funeral or burial rite.

Bereavement support

In hospice care, involvement with the family doesn't end when the patient dies. Organizations that provide end-of-life care must provide bereavement support for up to 1 year after the patient's death. Bereavement counselors contact survivors soon after the patient's death. This initial contact gives survivors the opportunity to retell their stories to someone they feel can understand without questioning. Further contacts allow the survivors to gradually place the death in the context of their ongoing life. The bereavement counselor can also assess how the family is doing socially, physically, and financially, and make referrals if needed. Family members may or may not avail themselves of bereavement services in the form of letters, telephone contact, and individual or group support sessions.

The bereavement group may evolve into another support system. Even if family members live in a different state than the patient, they can go to their local hospice and receive bereavement support and follow-up services. Bereavement support is also available through mental health professionals. The hospice bereavement coordinator can identify survivors who need extra psychological help.

Counseling is also available for children who have lost a parent, sibling, grandparent, or peer. Day- or week-long camps for surviving children are held annually by hospices nationwide. Also, many school counselors work with families of children affected by the death of someone close to them. School counselors uncomfortable working with bereaved children may prefer to contact their local hospice and ask a bereavement counselor to work with the child.

Community support

Resources are available outside the palliative care team and the main caregivers as well. Some are community based and serve a larger population, but may be accessed with the assistance of the hospice social worker. (See *Community resources in end-of-life care.*)

Community resources in end-of-life care

Some of the resources listed below serve any patient in need with little proof of eligibility. Some, like the American Cancer Society's one-time payment program for cancer patients in financial need, and the pharmaceutical programs for free drugs, require special paperwork and physician verification to provide benefits. The social worker on the palliative care team can help families obtain local services through these agencies.

- American Cancer Society
- Area Agency on Aging
- Energy companies
- Local churches
- Meals on Wheels

- Pharmaceutical companies
- Private charities
- Private nursing services
- Salvation Army
- Support groups

With the electronic age, hospice and palliative care have been able to disseminate valuable information to patients, families, organizations and professionals in all walks of life. Many resources are available via the Internet and can be accessed from home. (See *Using the Internet for support,* pages 220 and 221.) These sites can give assurance that the patient or caregiver is not alone. Many of them host chat rooms for patients or caregivers as well as providing up-to-date information.

Another source of support may be the extended family and friends of the patient or caregiver. For example, a spouse caring for a partner may ask for help from grown children. Single adults may eventually need help from their parents. Young families may call upon their siblings and parents. The extended family of relatives, friends, and neighbors may help with shopping, making a meal, providing transportation, sitting with a patient who can no longer be left alone, and phoning regularly to listen and support.

At times, you may find that many people are interested in helping but the patient or caregiver doesn't know how to accept help, perhaps having always been in the helper role before. If that happens, work with family members to help them recognize their value as unique individuals regardless of their present need, and encourage them to allow their loved ones the opportunity of this final gift of caring.

Using the Internet for support

Here are some examples of Internet sites patients and families can investigate for support and links to additional support and services.

Organization	Web address
Compassionate Friends	www.compassionatefriends.org
Dougy Center for Grieving Children and Families	www.dougy.org
Hospice Foundation of America	www.hospicefoundation.org
Tragedy Assistance Program for Survivors	www.taps.org
National Hospice and Palliative Care Organization	www.nhpco.org
	www.caringinfo.org
American Cancer Society	www.cancer.org
American Heart Association	www.americanheart.org
COPD International	www.copd-international.com
Alzheimer's Association	www.alz.org
ALS Association	www.alsa.org
Family Caregiving 101	www.familycaregiving101.org

Mission

To help families move toward positive resolution of grief after the death of a child of any age and to provide information to help others be supportive

Through the National Center for Grieving Children and Families, to provide support and training locally, nationally, and internationally to individuals and organizations seeking to assist children in grief

To help those who cope personally or professionally with terminal illness, death, and the process of grief and bereavement

To provide comfort and support to American armed forces' families dealing with the death of a loved one through peer support, crisis intervention, casework, grief and trauma resources and information, seminars, camps, and an on-line chat group

To lead and mobilize social change for improved care at the end of life

Site for patients and families

To eliminate cancer as a major health problem by preventing cancer, saving lives, and diminishing suffering from cancer through research, education, advocacy, and service

To reduce disability and death from cardiovascular diseases and stroke

To provide information and interactive support for COPD patients, caregivers, families and concerned individuals

To eliminate Alzheimer's disease through the advancement of research; to provide and enhance care and support for all affected; to reduce the risk of dementia through the promotion of brain health

To find a cure for and improve living with amyotrophic lateral sclerosis

To recognize, support, and advise family caregivers

16 | When death nears

Regardless of the setting in which a patient's death occurs, your main goal as death approaches is to normalize the process for the patient and the family, thus ensuring the best possible transition. Knowing what to expect will help patients and their loved ones make decisions about how to help, who should provide care, where care should be provided, and what steps the patient and family can take to help the patient die at peace.

Each patient is unique. Each family is unique. Each dying person and family experiences the journey to the end of life with a specific set of psychological, spiritual, cultural, and family issues. Caring for terminally ill patients requires flexibility, a patient-centered approach, and an ability to compassionately listen and facilitate, meeting the patient's needs and also supporting the family. As Dame Cicely Saunders, the founder of the modern-day hospice movement, has said, "How people die remains in the memories of those who live on."

The palliative care team, often mainly the nurses, must help the family and caregivers find a level of comfort with their roles and provide them with the knowledge and support they need to achieve the goals of care as set out by the dying person. Naturally, these goals will shift and change in the process, as will the roles of the family and the health care team.

Setting the stage

Sharing the signs and symptoms of approaching death in a gentle and timely manner will help the patient and family cope with the process. (See *Signs and symptoms of approaching death*.) Often, family members will notice changes but won't understand the significance of what they're seeing.

Signs and symptoms of approaching death

Body system	Signs and symptoms
Respiratory	▪ Shortness of breath ▪ Cough ▪ Mucus production
Gastrointestinal	▪ Nausea and vomiting ▪ Sore mouth ▪ Poor appetite and weight loss ▪ Constipation and diarrhea
Musculoskeletal	▪ Obvious deterioration ▪ Weakness ▪ Sluggishness, lethargy, lack of energy ▪ Muscle twitching, especially in limbs
Skin	▪ Irritation or dryness ▪ Pressure areas that appear quickly ▪ Pressure sores possible ▪ Jaundiced, pale, or gray color ▪ Loose skin from weight loss ▪ Aversion to touch, including blankets
Genitourinary	▪ Urinary tract infections ▪ Foul smelling, cloudy, or concentrated urine ▪ Bladder spasms ▪ Urine retention
Cardiac	▪ Edema of the limbs and sacral area possible ▪ Abdominal swelling possible
Neuropsychological	▪ Less engaged in family activities ▪ Less concerned with talking or hearing about family news ▪ More focused on personal needs and comfort ▪ Less ability to empathize with others' needs or feelings ▪ Possible agitation with unclear cause, including picking at covers or clothes

Teaching during this time can relieve a great deal of stress and help the family determine if sufficient resources are in place for them as the patient's needs change. This is also a time for spiritual conversations with the family and the patient, if he's able, to help them work toward meaningful closure.

Often, a dying person seems to withdraw and become more narrowly focused and introspective. Some retire into a bedroom; others bring their bed out into the living room. Either place then becomes the center of the household.

While the patient's still able, this may become the time for a life review, finding meaning in life, and making peace. This process can be profound. Family members and caregivers commonly need a reminder that simply sitting and listening may, at this time, be the most important and appreciated role that they have. Many books have been written about the final gifts that may be gathered at this time; recommending some to the family might be greatly helpful and appreciated.

Providing information

As you see the patient's death coming nearer, it's crucial to be proactive in telling family and caregivers what to expect. Now is the time to prepare families, in general, for the probable course of the patient's death. Each disease has specific symptoms to explain. Some families want everything explained at once; some prefer small amounts of information over time. Similarly, some members of the family may be designated to receive and interpret information, whereas others prefer not to hear the news directly. It may be helpful to have written information or checklists available. The importance of building rapport with the patient's support system and assessing the family dynamics can't be overstated. By exploring these dynamics, the team can effectively help the family and caregivers find and feel comfortable in their roles.

Estimating time

It's very common, almost universal, for patients and family members to ask how much time is left. Most research with bereaved families suggests that it's helpful for them to know what to expect and when to expect it. The best course is to give the family a range based on how the patient is doing at the present time and your experience with other patients in similar circumstances. Express the range as weeks to months, days to weeks, hours to days.

This may also be a good time to explain that things can change very quickly and, if there's anything that's important for them to accomplish before their loved dies, it may be wise to do it sooner than later. Explore whether there's someone else the patient may want to see or speak to or an event the patient may be waiting for. A family member may need to assume the role of facilitating these arrangements for the dying person.

A similar discussion might be centered on how each person might feel if the death happened when they weren't present. Some family members wish to be present and some don't. (See *Missing the moment.*) Talking about these issues ahead of time helps to prevent regrets later.

EXPERT INSIGHTS

Missing the moment

Recently, a dying patient's two adult daughters took turns staying at their mother's bedside for 3 days, around the clock. On the fourth day, they took a short break together — and that's when their mother died. Now one daughter feels tremendous regret that "Mama died alone," even though I assured them that two nurses were present and that their mother died peacefully. What more can I do? — A.F., Conn.

Try having a sensitive discussion with this patient's daughters. When this situation came up for me recently, I started by finding a private setting for a quiet talk. I gathered the grieving children and the nurses who were at their mother's bedside. I asked the nurses to recount again how peaceful and comfortable their mother was — "just like she's been with you throughout your lovely vigil."

The patient's daughter asked if her mother regained consciousness and asked for her children. "No," said one of the nurses, "she remained still and peaceful. Joanne and I sat quietly with her after we turned her and moistened her lips."

Then I offered a few little anecdotes to illustrate how often we see this happen. "Once another daughter in a similar situation kept watch over her mother for several days. She went home for a quick shower and change of clothes. Shortly after she left the room, her dear mother died. Another patient waited until his wife stepped into the restroom and then died."

If I were in your shoes, I'd take the hands of both daughters, who may be crying by now, and share the following observation: "I've come to believe that if the patient wants family to be present at the last breath they will be, and if she doesn't, they won't."

This may lead them to ask, "But why wouldn't Mama want us with her at the end?"

Having observed thousands of deaths, I'm convinced that we fully participate in how and where and when we leave the planet. Simply remind them that dying is a spiritual experience — and quite an intimate one. Encourage them not to take their mother's choice personally: "She needed to do this in her own way and time."

Acknowledge the fine job that they did in keeping vigil. And remind them, very gently, that this wasn't about them. When it's their turn, they'll understand and do it their own way too.

— JOY UFEMA, RN, MS

The final days

As the signs of approaching death progress, if the patient is in hospice, the team typically increases nursing and home health aide visits to assist the family with care. Gradually, it will become apparent that the patient may have only days to live. (See *Death within days.*) Family members probably will be talking about how he's changing.

At this stage, the patient typically is confined to bed and is profoundly weak. He needs complete bed care and can't participate at all in his own care. He's probably pale and gaunt, with longer and longer periods of somnolence. It's very difficult for him to concentrate or pay attention, and he may be disoriented to time and place. He's less and less interested in food and has trouble swallowing food, fluids, and oral medications.

To ease the patient's final days, prepare to address common developments—both with the patient and the family.

Decreasing food and fluids

Appetite decreases at this time, as does enjoyment of food. This can be a very stressful change for loved ones because, for many people, food is a way to express love and forms the centerpiece of celebrations and happy memories. It isn't unusual for a dying patient to request his favorite dish, only to be unable to eat it or uninterested in eating it when it arrives. Gently explain that hunger decreases through the dying process. Reassure worried family members that the patient isn't starving to death and that the body doesn't need nourishment at this time. Discussing this ahead of time may reduce feelings of rejection or despair that caregivers might otherwise feel.

If swallowing becomes difficult, gently point out to family and caregivers that pushing fluids may cause the patient to choke. Show them how to give small amounts of fluid with a syringe to help keep the patient comfortable. Many family members worry that their loved one is thirsty as fluid intake decreases. Explain that most experts feel that dehydration in the last hours of life causes no distress and may actually stimulate the release of endorphins and anesthetic compounds that promote the patient's sense of well-being.

Family members also may ask you whether the patient should receive intravenous fluids. Explain that, although giving I.V. fluids may help certain symptoms, it also may overload the body with fluids that can't be accommodated, thus causing painful edema and increasing shortness of breath. Instead, show family members how to provide mouth care (mouth swabs, ice chips, or both) to prevent drying and promote comfort for their loved one. This loving task can be helpful both for the patient and for the family member who feels the need to do something.

Death within days

As a patient comes within days of death, you may notice evidence of several changes, including changes in muscle tone, circulation, vital signs, senses, and level of consciousness.

Change	Evidence
Loss of muscle tone	▪ Relaxation of facial muscles ▪ Trouble swallowing ▪ Gradual loss of gag reflex ▪ Decreased gastrointestinal activity ▪ Possible urinary and fecal incontinence from relaxation of sphincters ▪ Assistance needed to move in bed and perform all activities of daily living ▪ Increased sleeping
Slowing of circulation	▪ Reduced skin sensation ▪ Mottling of limbs, nail beds, ears, and nose ▪ Cold limbs, feet, hands, ears, and nose ▪ Possible increased edema in the lower legs or sacum ▪ Diaphoresis
Altered vital signs	▪ Weaker pulse that may be rapid or irregular ▪ Lower blood pressure ▪ Rapid, shallow, irregular, or slower breathing ▪ Possible increased temperature
Sensory impairment	▪ Blurred vision ▪ Decreased senses of taste and smell (probable continued sense of hearing)
Altered level of consciousness	▪ Variable consciousness, from alert to drowsy to comatose ▪ Decreased responsiveness ▪ Possible decreased pain sensation ▪ Possible decreased mental function and trouble with speech ▪ Possible withdrawal in preparation for leaving ▪ Possible hallucinations or visions

Increasing sleep

Decreasing awareness and increasing periods of sleeping may seem to the family as though the patient is giving up. Help them understand that these changes are normal, and urge them to give the patient permission to rest.

As death nears, the patient may lie utterly still in bed. If needed, reassure the family that this is normal and okay. Explain, however, that this inactivity may lead to joint stiffness and discomfort and an increased risk of pressure areas, especially over bony prominences. Teach strategies for positioning and supporting the patient with pillows and padding, emphasizing less frequent turning and moving, which will become increasingly uncomfortable. If needed, provide prophylactic pain control before turning the patient.

Changing circulation

The family also may notice changes in the patient's body temperature as death approaches. His hands and feet may feel very cold one minute and then become warm again. One hand may feel cold and the other warm. The skin may become mottled on the limbs, around the mouth and nose, and on dependent parts of the body. If you don't explain these changes ahead of time, family members could be alarmed when they turn the patient and see what appears to be bruising on his back or buttocks, for instance. Explain that these marks stem from circulatory changes and that the patient isn't aware of them.

Altered breathing

One of the most common symptoms of impending death is a change in breathing pattern to Cheyne-Stokes respirations. This is also one of the most distressing symptoms for family and caregivers. Early in the process, when the patient's breathing is becoming shallower, explain that Cheyne-Stokes respirations probably will develop. Reassure the family that this is a normal end-stage breathing pattern and that the dying person isn't aware of it or distressed by it. Another distressing symptom is the noisy, gurgling breathing commonly known as a death rattle. This change is a good predictor that death is near. One study gives a median time of 16 hours from the start of the death rattle to the patient's death.

Family and caregivers may worry that the dying person is drowning and may ask if suctioning would help. Teach family members that the noisy breathing is the sound of air moving over secretions that the dying person can no longer clear or swallow. Explain that the dying person isn't aware of or struggling with this symptom. Often, a simple change of position will relieve the sound.

Usually, suctioning doesn't help because the secretions are beyond the reach of the suction catheter. What's more, frequent suctioning would be disturbing to the patient — more disturbing than the noisy breathing.

ALERT
If the patient appears distressed or the family is very distressed, obtain an order for a drug to help reduce the secretions.

Incontinence

Another fear often expressed by patients, families, and caregivers is a loss of bowel and bladder control in the final stages of dying. For this issue, reassurance may need to be more than verbal. Keep appropriate supplies available in case they're needed, and teach the most appropriate care provider how to use them.

This is a role that many family members may not be able to handle, or they may feel that their loved one would not feel comfortable with them providing this care. Exploring this ahead of time and planning for the appropriate person or provider will help prevent crisis calls or at least provide the family with a plan of action should it be needed.

If urinary incontinence is a problem, an indwelling catheter can be helpful. However, if urine output is minimal, absorbent padding and protection is often sufficient. Family members probably won't know that decreased fluid intake and kidney function will lead to darker, more concentrated urine. Warning the family and caregivers about the darker color of urine will help to relieve their distress when they see it for the first time.

Cachexia

With advanced wasting, the patient loses fat pads, subcutaneous tissue, and muscle mass. The cachectic appearance of their loved one can cause distress in the caregivers. The patient's eyes may stay open or partly open, and attempts to keep them closed will be unsuccessful. Lax muscles also may be the reason for a perpetually open mouth and noisy mouth breathing. Explain why this happens, and teach the family how to maintain moisture, such as using artificial tears. Doing so may give the family and caregivers comfort and help them in affirming their role in providing quality care for their dying loved one.

Agitation

Agitated delirium may be the first indication of a difficult road to death instead of the peaceful progression that everyone would prefer. If your patient becomes restless or confused, thoroughly assess whether there's a simple, treatable cause. Is the restlessness from urine retention that could be remedied with an indwelling catheter? Could it be increasing or uncontrolled pain?

Reassure the family that it's unusual for uncontrolled pain to develop in the late stages of dying but that there are signs to watch for and strategies for treatment. When discussing pain control in the terminal stages, explain to or remind the family and caregivers that the patient's kidneys and liver are no longer functioning well and that drugs, especially opioids, can accumulate and cause symptoms such as increasing agitation and muscle jerking (myoclonus). If these symptoms don't occur, pain medication usually continues at its previous level in the last hours of life.

This discussion is especially important if family members feel that the patient might wake up and talk if only the pain medication were stopped. Gently remind them about the goals of palliative care and the need to protect the patient's comfort and quality of life.

Altered senses

When death is hours to minutes away, the patient may progress to a semi-comatose and then to a comatose state. (See *When death is imminent.*) As communicating with their loved one becomes more difficult, caregivers' stress levels and anxiety increase. Explain to family and caregivers that the change stems from organ functions shutting down. Reassure them that their loved one isn't as distressed by these changes as they, the observers, are. This is an opportunity to help them to define their roles in providing comfort and helping their loved one achieve his goals as death approaches.

The patient may lose visual acuity or may have an increased sensitivity to bright lights. Adjust the room lights to the patient's comfort level. Hearing is the last sense to fade; reassure family members that the patient can hear them. Urge them to continue talking softly and calmly to their dying loved one. This often is a time of story telling around the bedside and can be a time of laughter and reminiscence. Some family members may need reassurance that laughter and camaraderie at this time is perfectly acceptable. Also, encourage family members to touch the patient in a comforting manner, keeping in mind that touching may not be considered helpful in some cultures or families of origin.

This is also the time to stop nursing care activities that serve no further purpose. For example, family members may be frightened by seeing blood pressure numbers diminish or be only palpable. Explain to the patient and his family that important items such as pain and symptom control will be monitored but temperature, pulse, respirations, and blood pressure numbers are now secondary to the patient's comfort and spiritual and emotional status.

Nearing-death awareness

An increasing number of anecdotal reports suggest that dying people may have a nearing-death awareness. If family or caregivers haven't heard of this phenomenon, they may mistakenly think that the dying person is delirious or confused, and they may miss the opportunity to communicate with the patient on a very meaningful level. Instead, they may express fear or frustration.

The anecdotes typically recount the patient seeing or speaking to dead family or friends or talking about going on a trip or packing a bag. The pa-

When death is imminent

When a patient is within hours or minutes of dying, you'll observe these characteristics:

- large, fixed pupils
- inability to move
- faster, weaker pulse
- lower blood pressure
- Cheyne-Stokes respirations
- noisy breathing (commonly called the death rattle) from mucus in the throat
- inability or minimal ability to speak.

tient may ask for something or someone as a means to facilitate a peaceful death. Encourage the family to listen carefully during this time and help decipher these messages. Explain that they can ask the patient about messages they don't understand but shouldn't contradict or argue with him. When they're unsure what to say, they can acknowledge that they don't understand but will keep trying, or they may simply say nothing and just be present with the patient.

The moment of death

The moment of death is not often a crisis of distress; for most, the suffering is over before they die. Usually there's a period of calm, and few are aware of the advent of their own death.

Family members may ask how to know when their loved one has died. (See *Clinical signs of death*, page 232.) People who have never seen a person at the moment of death can be frightened or unsure of themselves in addition to facing the reality that the loved one is really gone. Others are comfortable at this moment and able to make calls calmly, putting aside their emotions until the patient leaves the house or facility for the last time. You and other members of the team can prepare the family for this moment based on their questions and needs. Encourage them to call the staff at any time for help or to assist at the time of death.

Indeed, throughout the process of the patient's dying, the patient, family, and caregivers will need continuing education and support. Participating in the experience of another's death makes one aware of his own mortality. Effective, holistic care providers, whether family or professional, are comfortable with their own mortality and able to think and talk about both the patient's death and their own.

Clinical signs of death

- No response to external stimuli
- No muscular movement
- No reflexes
- No breathing
- No pulse
- No eye response

Family and caregiver involvement in actual hands-on care will vary with the setting. Obviously, if a patient's preference is to die at home, the family will be more involved in providing physical care and making care decisions. In an acute care setting, the actual care may fall to the staff, but the comfort measures and family roles remain and should be addressed when providing information to the family. The same applies in a skilled nursing facility. This is considered the dying person's home. Even if the staff is the only "family" available to provide care, family comfort and support roles still must be considered.

Caring for a dying person can be difficult and exhausting, both mentally and physically. Thus, a solid support system should be in place to provide the education and guidance needed through the process of dying and on into bereavement. Caring for a loved one at this stage of life can give a profound sense of satisfaction to caregivers. The support and assistance you provide can help the patient and family negotiate the difficult final chapter of life and is the memory that will live on in the minds of loved ones and caregivers. Compassion turns ordinary care into extraordinary care, which will greatly ease the distress and discomfort of dying patients and their loved ones.

Bereavement care 17

It's the responsibility of helping professions such as physicians, nurses, and related professionals to provide care not only to dying patients but to bereaved survivors. (See *Nursing responsibilities in bereavement care*, page 234.) The care needed may vary with the type of grief response survivors have, their ability to work through their grief, their age, and their family environment.

Recognizing grief

Although any perceived loss can cause some level of grief, the loss of a loved one can bring with it the most intense grief response. This intense reaction may be a normal grief response or it may reflect a complicated grief response.

Normal grief

A normal grief response affects all aspects of a person's being, including physical, cognitive, emotional, behavioral, and spiritual. Some or all of these responses may occur simultaneously. (See *Characteristics of grief responses*, page 235.)

Physically, bereaved persons are at risk for new illness or worsening of existing illness during the first year after experiencing a loss. Cognitively, no matter how much the death is expected, when it occurs, family members experience shock and disbelief. This will be more pronounced when someone dies suddenly. People may report seeing the deceased person.

Emotional acceptance takes time. When the death is acknowledged cognitively, the bereaved person opens his emotions to the pain. The aware-

---

Nursing responsibilities in bereavement care

■ Provide information and education with sensitivity to what people want to know.
■ Provide emotional support.
■ Recognize abnormal bereavement reactions.
■ Manage appropriate referrals to mental health resources.
■ Legitimize the occurrence of the death.

---

ness of loss may occur in incremental amounts as the person can endure it. The bereaved person may imagine what he might have done to prevent the death. Guilt may be intense if the bereaved person was indirectly involved in the death of the family member. The sadness may be broken at times but returns quickly with reminders of the deceased person, such as sorting the person's clothes or hearing the person's favorite song.

Behaviorally, daily functioning returns gradually after the initial shock of the death. The bereaved person must take care of the funeral or burial and adjust to the role changes brought about by the death of a family member. Behaviors that are destructive to self or others or involve substance abuse are maladaptive but not unusual.

Spiritual beliefs about death and life after death differ and will affect the way each person grieves. A family's religion and culture may prescribe certain acts and behaviors after a death, but individual family members may or may not hold those beliefs.

Complicated grief

Some people have abnormal—also known as complicated—grief responses. These can stem from various internal and external factors, including the circumstances of the death and the person's relationship with the deceased. The bereaved person may have had an ambivalent relationship with the deceased before death. The survivor may have unexpressed hostility toward the deceased. In this case, the survivor is likely to feel anger and guilt, which inhibit grief.

Another type of ambivalent relationship is a highly narcissistic one in which the deceased is seen as an extension of the surviving family member. A person grieving a death in a highly dependent relationship has lost the source of that dependency and will experience a change in self-image.

Characteristics of grief responses

Type of response	Characteristics
Physical	Anorexia Dry mouth Fatigue Feelings of choking Frequent sighing GI disturbances Headaches Problems sleeping Shortness of breath Tightness in the throat or chest Weakness
Cognitive	Confusion Denial Disbelief Preoccupation with the image of the deceased Shock Trouble concentrating Visual illusions
Emotional	Anger Fears of being crazy Feelings of being out of control Feelings of guilt Sadness Searching for the deceased Yearning
Behavioral	Crying Disorganized activity Disrupted activities of daily living Eating disturbances Excessive work Loss of interest in activities Quick temper Restlessness
Spiritual	Anger at God Disrupted belief in God Guilt Questioning of the meaning of life and death Reinforcement of beliefs

Characteristics of complicated grief reactions

Type of complicated grief	Characteristics
Delayed	■ Feelings related to the loss are unexpressed until a later loss. ■ Feelings may arise in response to another person's loss.
Exaggerated	■ Response is more intense than usual. ■ Response is out of proportion to the loss. ■ Affected person is disabled by clinical depression or other psychiatric diagnosis.
Chronic	■ Reaction is unusually long. ■ Reaction never reaches a resolution.
Masked	■ Feelings aren't expressed overtly. ■ Feelings are expressed as physical symptoms or maladaptive behavior. ■ Survivor has no recognition that symptoms or behaviors are related to loss. ■ Survivor may feel symptoms of deceased person's illness.

Feelings of helplessness may overwhelm the person's ability to experience and work through intense feelings of grief.

Many circumstantial factors may lead to complicated grief. Among them are uncertain losses, such as a soldier missing in action. The bereaved are never sure that the person is really dead. Multiple losses, such as those that occur in disasters, airplane crashes, earthquakes, hurricanes, and fires leave bereaved family members with bereavement overload after losing several family members, their home, and their life as they once knew it. Those with complicated grief after one loss will have trouble resolving later losses.

Survivors of someone who has committed suicide may be less likely to discuss their loved one's death from fear of the social stigma. This creates a conspiracy of silence that deprives the survivors of the social support that's normally a part of bereavement. The survivor who discovered the body of the deceased may be left with terrible memories.

Another circumstance that reduces support for the bereaved is a socially negated loss, such as abortion. The decision to abort is usually made in isolation, and the woman's family isn't involved. Social isolation itself can complicate grieving. People move around the country, and many live without close proximity to extended family. When a family member dies, the survivor may have no one who even knew the deceased.

Recognizing complicated grief is difficult because normal grief responses are very intense. In complicated grief, the survivor's grief intensifies to the point of overwhelm, and the person may resort to maladaptive behaviors. The difference between normal grief and complicated grief isn't the presence of a symptom but its intensity and duration. (See *Characteristics of complicated grief reactions.*)

Bereaved individuals with complicated grief reactions should be referred for counseling. Resources for referrals of complicated grief should be readily available in agencies and facilities where families may suffer the loss of a family member.

Caring for individuals

When caring for a bereaved person — a person in mourning — one way to frame the process is by viewing successful bereavement as the completion of certain tasks. Such tasks may include accepting the reality of the person's death, continuing to work through the pain, adjusting to the new environment and way of life, and making the emotional shift that allows the person to move on.

Accepting reality

Even when death is expected, survivors must come to terms with the reality that death has occurred. The opposite of accepting the reality is denial of the loss or of the meaning of the loss. (See *Accepting the reality of death,* page 238.)

You can help surviving family members begin to accept reality. Although no one should be forced to view a body, seeing the deceased's body after death may be important in helping close family members acknowledge the death and begin to form tolerable memories of the death of their loved one.

If the death resulted from trauma, the emergency department team shouldn't completely remove all evidence of physical intervention, so survivors can see the efforts made to save their loved one's life. However, evidence that survivors might find horrifying should be removed so the family can see their loved one without the shock of seeing blood and other signs of suffering.

After a sudden death, it's helpful if two people with authority are present to break the news. If possible, they should stay to share the subsequent reactions of the survivors. The sensitivity (or lack of it) of professionals in telling the family members the bad news will be remembered long after the event and may be relived repeatedly as the survivor grieves the loss.

Accepting the reality of death

You can help a bereaved person accept the reality of a loved one's death by providing these services.

- Facilitate the viewing of the body.
- Present bad news with sensitivity.
- Use active listening.
- Acknowledge the person's anger.

Active listening will help grieving people express their emotions and begin to work through the pain of grief. The grieving person will repeat the story of the loss over and over. Repetition is an effort to absorb the reality of the loss, to believe in what has happened. Ask the bereaved person what happened or later in the process ask what the funeral was like. Letting the person repeat the story, using the name of the deceased and the word *death* instead of a euphemism, helps them accept the reality of the loss.

Anger isn't uncommon after a loss and may be directed toward helping professionals. Don't take it personally. Acknowledging the survivor's anger will be perceived as support. Defensive statements or reasoning will be perceived as confrontation and may increase the bereaved person's anger. Acting out in an aggressive manner is unacceptable, however, and needs immediate intervention with help from security or police. Survivors who become violent toward others or themselves early after the death should be referred for immediate intervention. Drug and alcohol abuse is maladaptive as well.

Working through pain

Nurses can play an important role in helping the bereaved to complete the task of getting through the pain of grief. (See *Working through the pain of grief.*)

Immediately after a death, your quiet presence can comfort the family survivors. Many nurses, accustomed to always doing something, underestimate the value of presence. Simply stand by and witness the survivors' emotional expressions without trying to fix them. Grief is painful and necessary. Being there is a form of empathy and is crucial to a supportive relationship during the mourning process.

Tears and sadness on your part are fine, if genuine. Real emotions demonstrate to the bereaved that you valued their loved one and reinforce the reality of the loss. However, avoid expressing emotions that require comfort by the bereaved person or family.

Grieving people often are frightened of their strong feelings and the inability to think and concentrate. They fear they are going crazy and that

Working through the pain of grief

You can help a bereaved person work through his grief by providing these services.
- Maintain a quiet presence.
- Reassure the person that strong grief responses are normal.
- Explain why medications, such as antidepressants, probably won't help.
- Provide information as needed, including about support services.

they'll never be free of pain. Normalizing these responses to grief can be helpful when applied appropriately. Tell them that intense feelings and lack of concentration, though very painful, are experienced by many people after a significant loss. This information can reduce their feeling out of control and address their fears about feeling crazy. Be careful, however, that your efforts to normalize their feelings don't minimize them instead. Also, don't try to normalize their emotions by saying, "I know how you feel." Instead, explain that others who are grieving have reported these painful responses.

Some people gain emotional strength and insights from writing. For those who do, suggest writing in a journal or writing a letter. Writing can be an outlet for intense emotions. Reading may help as well. Many books are available that address personal responses to illness and grief. Recommend them to those who are interested. If someone is having difficulty dealing with his grief, help him find support. Many organizations offer help to grieving people. (See *Resources for dealing with grief,* pages 240 and 241.)

Most authorities discourage the use of medication, particularly antidepressants, for those in bereavement. One reason is the length of time needed for these drugs to take effect. Another is that these drugs may be dangerous for people who might consider suicide. Tranquilizers may be used in complicated grief, particularly for a person already taking psychotropic drugs for mental illness. These drugs aren't appropriate in normal grief, where the tranquilized person may lose the opportunity to express feelings early after the loss, when family, friends, and supportive professionals are present. Plus, the tranquilizer eventually will wear off, usually after the funeral when extended family and friends have moved back into their own lives. Finally, in a normal grief response, tranquilizers may reinforce latent substance abuse and delay normal grief responses.

Provide whatever information the family needs to get through the funeral and bereavement. This begins by explaining all procedures provided by your agency that are related to the deceased. Provide information about support groups in the area that address the appropriate type of loss (parental

Resources for dealing with grief

Organization	Web address
AARP	www.aarp.org/families/grief
American Foundation for Suicide Prevention	www.afsp.org
Association for Death Education and Counseling	www.adec.org
Centering Corporation	www.centeringcorp.com/catalog/
Compassionate Friends	www.compassionatefriends.org
Dougy Center for Grieving Children and Families	www.dougy.org
Hospice Foundation of America	www.hospicefoundation.org
National Hospice and Palliative Care Organization	www.nhpco.org
National Sudden Infant Death Syndrome Center	www.sidscenter.org

loss, child loss). Provide written information or pamphlets for the family to keep. They may not be interested in reading the information now but will refer to it later when they're ready.

Adjusting to the environment

Adjusting to a world without the deceased will take a long time—months to years. (See *Adjusting to the environment of loss*, page 242.) The role the deceased occupied in the family will influence the kinds of adjustments that must be made. You can facilitate the bereaved person's ability to live without the deceased by helping the person address these role changes. For example, a widow who has never made decisions on her own must learn the role of decision-maker that her spouse once filled. A problem-solving approach, familiar to nurses, is useful here. Help the widow focus on and assess her decision-making abilities, and suggest groups or classes to assist

Description

Provides information, advocacy, and benefits to people age 50 and older

Educates professionals and the public about suicide and its prevention

Promotes excellence in death education, bereavement counseling, and care of the dying

Provides education and resources for the bereaved through a catalog containing many books specific to grief after all types of losses

Offers support groups for bereaved parents

Provides support and training locally, nationally, and internationally to individuals and organizations seeking to assist children and teens in their grief

Promotes hospice care and works to educate professionals and families in caregiving, terminal illness, loss, and bereavement

Provides educational programs, technical assistance, and public policy advocacy

Provides information services and technical assistance on sudden infant death syndrome and related topics

her. Meeting with other widows offers the opportunity for learning and sharing.

Counsel the newly bereaved to postpone making life-changing decisions, such as selling a house, moving to a new city, or changing jobs or careers. Impulsive life-changing decisions may reflect an urge to run away from the pain of grief. Often, running away removes the bereaved person from her supportive environment and intensifies her social isolation.

If you have long-term contact with family survivors, continue to let them talk about their loss if they want to. The time after the funeral can be the most difficult. Often, after a few months, social supports related to the loss disappear as people go about their own lives, yet family survivors may still need to talk about their deceased family member and their grief experiences. Support is just as important in the later weeks of the mourning process. People in the bereaved person's life may avoid bringing up the topic because they fear making the person sad, yet the sadness is already there,

Adjusting to the environment of loss

You can help a bereaved person adjust to his changed environment
by providing these services.
- Facilitate the adjustment by addressing changes in family roles.
- Encourage the bereaved person to delay life-changing decisions.
- Offer emotional support by letting survivors talk about their feelings.
- Support the bereaved person in emotional relocation.

with few means of expression. Each person is different, though; be sensitive
to the survivor's need to talk or be silent about a loved one's death.

Grief for survivors resurfaces on holidays and anniversaries after a death.
This is a normal reaction, and family members should be told to expect it.
Tell family members that planning a visit to the cemetery or an activity to
express their grief is better than avoiding the emotions.

Allowing emotional relocation

To resolve a loss over time, the bereaved doesn't forget the deceased or the
grief but eventually puts the loss into a life perspective. A bereaved spouse
creates a new relationship in his mind with the deceased spouse. The memories will always remain and become integrated into the bereaved's personality. Eventually, the grief work reaches a point that the bereaved person is
ready to invest emotionally in a new relationship or to move on with his
life without the deceased person as a living part of it. Worden calls this
emotional relocation. Reminiscing is one method a bereaved person can
use to gradually divest the emotional energy attached to the deceased.

A new relationship can never replace the one that was lost. The new person in a relationship with the bereaved person must be recognized as an individual for the new relationship to work. Helping with this task can take
the form of encouraging memorials, listening to reminiscence, and acknowledging and accepting new relationships while continuing to respect
the memory of the deceased.

Caring for children

Like adults, children experience highly individualized grief responses.
They're influenced by some of the same factors as adult grief, such as age,
personality, previous experience with death, and relationship with the deceased. However, children are less able than adults to label their emotions,

and their response to loss isn't continuous. A child's grief may appear inter-mittent. He may be sad one minute and outside laughing and playing the next minute.

A child's grief is influenced most by his developmental stage and cognitive ability to understand the permanence of the loss. (See *How children view death*, page 244.) A child's grief lasts longer than adult grief because children need to work through the loss at each subsequent developmental stage. Children may not be able to identify their emotions, and they're likely to act out their feelings of grief as misbehavior.

Developmental guide

Infants and small children benefit from additional nurturing after a death in the family. Infants should be held often. They benefit from establishing and following a schedule for their care. During the acute stage of their grief, parents bereaved from the death of a child may have trouble providing this care to a surviving child. An extended relative or grandparent may need to help.

Three major themes in the grief responses of children are important to their care: Did they cause the death to happen, is it going to happen to them, and who is going to take care of them? Interventions designed to help children must address these issues.

Children in the stage of magical thinking believe that wishing something may make it so. If they were upset with the deceased person before death, they may believe their thoughts caused the death. They may never say this but continue to harbor the guilt. Intervene proactively by telling a child that nothing he thought or did caused the loved one to die. If a sibling died, the child may fear that he'll die soon, too. Reassure the child that he'll be all right.

Children depend on their parents or nurturing adults for their welfare, and they fear the loss of caretakers when a family member dies. They worry about who will take care of them. To make matters worse, after a death in the family, parents may shut children out of the rituals and hide their own emotional responses. Children who don't see their parents cry don't learn to deal with death openly. Consequently, they suffer their own grief alone. They may believe their parents didn't care about the death, which increases the risk of complicated grief.

Clear and simple

Explain a death clearly and simply to a child. Base the level of detail on the child's developmental ability to comprehend the death. Children will ask questions for a long time after a death as they mature. These questions should be addressed honestly and directly. Their concerns for their own welfare and security should be addressed by parents, who should make sure children understand the information provided. Encourage parents to bring

How children view death

Age	Response to death
Infant	■ Doesn't recognize death ■ Senses the absence of a parent and the changed atmosphere of the home ■ May respond with irritability, crying, and changes in bowel and bladder patterns ■ May become listless and unresponsive if separated from a source of nurturance ■ May have physical changes, such as weight loss ■ May have sleeplessness and other signs of agitation in response to a bereaved parent's emotional responses
2 to 3 years	■ Confuses death with sleep ■ May fear going to bed or being separated from parents ■ Senses parents' emotional responses ■ May generalize distress into behavior problems
3 to 6 years	■ Sees death as reversible, a kind of sleep ■ May fear and resist going to sleep ■ Sees death as influenced and possibly caused by thinking ■ May assume guilt for the death but be unable to express the feeling verbally ■ May have eating and sleeping disturbances ■ May regress in behaviors
6 to 9 years	■ May understand death as permanent ■ May be curious about death and the dead person's body ■ May be frightened by the finality of death ■ May think of death as happening to others, especially elderly people ■ May become clingy, refusing to go to school, or aggressive and destructive rather than expressing sadness directly ■ May have exaggerated fears
9 and older	■ Views death as permanent ■ By age 12, views death as inevitable and universal, that it may happen to them ■ Expresses grief through mood swings, heightened emotions, and increased anxiety about their own possible death ■ May have sleep problems, changes in eating habits, and regressive or impulsive behaviors
Adolescent	■ Experiences grief similarly to adults ■ Tends to hide emotions ■ May develop intensified behaviors normal to adolescence, such as rebellion ■ May have an increased risk of promiscuity and drug abuse

up the topic. One way to bring up the topic of death with children is to use one of the many story books written for children about death.

When talking with children, it's important to use the correct language, such as death and cancer. Avoid describing death as sleeping or passing because children will be confused and more fearful. Make sure you adhere to the cultural practices of the child's family.

Children should be included in funerals and memorials for loved ones but should never be forced to attend them. A full explanation of what will occur should be given in advance of the service. If the parents are too busy to pay close attention to the child, it's helpful to ask another responsible adult to care for the grieving child during the funeral.

Encourage a parent to contact the child's teacher after a death in the family. The teacher should be informed about the child's situation so the teacher can be sensitive to the child's grief and any behavioral reactions. The child also can be prepared ahead of time for questions from school mates. Peer pressure is especially important to adolescents and can provide a basis for intervention if there's a bereavement peer support group available.

Caring for families

The death of a family member is a crisis not only for individuals but for the family as a unit. The family will react in ways that reflect the underlying characteristics of the family, including cultural mandates, the current phase of the family life cycle, existing stressors, and the members' ability to communicate openly and provide emotional support for each other. Interventions on behalf of the family unit facilitate open communication and unity during bereavement.

Funerals, rituals, and memorials provide traditional methods of communication and serve the survivors' needs to reinforce the finality of the death in their extended family community and their culture. (See *Suggestions for bereaved patients and families*, page 246.) Publication of the death brings public acknowledgment and subsequent community support. Funerals, rituals, and memorial services bring together a supportive network in which the bereaved can talk about the deceased. If you have long-term professional connections to the deceased person, it's fine for you to attend services for your own sense of closure and to support the survivors.

Cultural sensitivity

The opportunity for intervention in family bereavement presents itself first when the family member is dying. Cultural and religious issues may dictate rituals around the death and how the body of the deceased is handled. Grief

---

Suggestions for bereaved patients and families

- Give yourself time to grieve.
- Expect intense feelings.
- Talk with others who have had a similar loss.
- Communicate with your family and friends.
- Postpone major decisions.
- Sleep and exercise.
- Try to eat healthy food.
- Avoid alcohol, drugs, and tobacco.
- Keep a journal or write a letter to the deceased.

- Prioritize daily activities.
- Lower your expectations for yourself.
- Read books or literature.
- Feed your spirit through a spiritual activity, such as church, or a peaceful place.
- Create a memorial book with photographs.
- Donate the deceased person's clothes to charity.
- Establish a memorial ritual of meaning to the family.

---

and mourning are common to all cultures. Ask about the family's customs and rituals surrounding death and grief. Ask survivors what shows respect for their loss and their family. Promote integration of the death and reinvestment in life for surviving family members by assessing and facilitating culturally relevant grieving practices.

Naturally, every family is unique. Even families with the same cultural background will hold different beliefs, customs, and preferences. Keeping that variation in mind, it may be possible to prepare yourself with a very general idea of how some cultures interact with death.

Black families

Black families constitute a large, varied group with many subcultures. For those who combine Western Christian beliefs with African beliefs, death and mourning practices commemorate the deceased through remembrance and celebration. In African culture, death is viewed as a transition signaling the end of one existence and the beginning of a new existence. Families gather in the home of the deceased and may travel great distances to support the family. The church family is a very important provider of spiritual support in this culture. Those who hold Islamic beliefs may have different rituals surrounding death.

Islamic families

Four main practices must be observed after the death of a believer. The specific methods and accessory rituals that accompany each of these basic practices vary from place to place and time to time. The members of the interdisciplinary team can best serve the patient by asking the family ahead of time what they need from the staff at the time of death and later when the funeral director is notified. The four basic practices are:

■ The body must be bathed by a Muslim, to physically clean it. This is called *ghusl*. There may be rules about who can perform this ritual and the use of certain scented oils or cleansing cloths.

■ The body must be wrapped from head to toe in clean, unornamented, cloth, called *kafan*. The cloth is usually white cotton and may be lightly scented. There may be specific rituals associated with this step.

■ The community gathers to pray over the body. This is called *salat*, and they recite the *Janazah* prayers.

■ The body must be buried in the ground, facing Mecca. The funeral procession is silent, without music or audible crying. If consistent with local laws, no casket is used. More prayers are said at the burial.

Quran theologians have studied Islamic law in regard to organ transplantation. In general, Muslims are instructed that they may not donate their organs for transplantation after their death, but can be a living donor of a kidney, blood, or bone marrow if a family member is at risk of death without such treatment.

Jewish families

There are many forms of Judaism that interpret Jewish law differently. Jewish death practices include rituals intended for the mourners and rituals for the care of the deceased person's body. Jewish law provides that the funeral and burial must occur as soon as possible after death, because the soul of the deceased begins to return to God immediately after death. In Jewish traditions, someone must watch over the body from the time of death until the burial.

The chevrah kadisha perform the traditional washing and dressing of the body, which is called *taharah*. The body is placed in a wood coffin that can have no metal parts. This facilitates the belief that all people are equal in death. Embalming is not done in the Jewish tradition. After the burial, the family returns home to begin sitting shivah for 7 days. During shivah, mourners contemplate their loss. After shivah, mourners continue in a 30-day period called shloshim. At the end of a 1-year mourning period, they may return to the graveyard for the first time, and they place a headstone on the grave. Bereaved individuals are traditionally cared for by their religious community.

Latino families

Latinos express their grief by crying openly. People close to the deceased are expected to express their grief openly. Friends and family offer them support and comfort. Latino men tend not to cry because they're expected to be strong. A bereaved Latino family is likely to follow Catholic religious traditions, to have an open-casket service, and to wear dark colors as a sign of mourning. Hugging or touching in this culture is considered a comforting gesture.

Hindu families

Hinduism describes a set of philosophies and cultures but has a uniform approach to death. Each birth is considered to be linked to previous births. Birth and death are part of a cycle in which Hindu people transcend to the liberation of the soul through the accumulation of good karmas or actions. When a Hindu person dies, before the next sunrise, the body is bathed, massaged in oil, and dressed in preparation for cremation. The body is not embalmed. Immediate cremation is believed to facilitate the soul's transition from this world to the next. The deceased isn't buried because doing so would keep the soul earthbound and confused. After cremation, several rituals are observed for the next 10 days. Family members eat only once per day of food cooked at home. Only on the 12th day does the family gather to honor and remember the deceased.

You must honor and facilitate each family's culturally prescribed rituals to the extent the family desires. For families without religious or culturally prescribed ritual, memorials can help the family members do something collectively to remember the deceased. For example, the family can choose to plant a tree as a living memorial for the deceased. Helping family members grieve includes respecting their cultural heritage. In the absence of a culturally prescribed tradition, encourage the family to decide how to commemorate the death in a way that's meaningful to them and that increases their support network.

Roles and relationships

Families change over time, and their roles change as they develop. The number of roles that must be reassigned and the importance of these roles to family functioning are central to the potential for family crisis. A family with young children has parents who are needed for all aspects of the children's welfare. The loss of one parent during this phase creates a greater need for role changes after the death than a family in which the children are adults and no longer dependent on their parents. Specific types of loss (parent, spouse, child) each have significant adjustment issues added to the grief process.

Death of a parent

Grief after the death of a parent will depend on the stage of the family life cycle. For a young child, loss of a parent may be devastating compared to the reaction of an independent adult who loses a parent. The role of the parent must be replaced or assumed entirely by the surviving parent. These role adjustments are required at a time when grief diminishes the capacity of the survivors. Intervention from social services may be needed for a child who loses a parent. The circumstances of the death, such as whether it was sudden and unexpected or followed a long-term illness, will affect the time needed to meet these demands.

Death of a spouse

The death of a spouse can be very traumatic. In addition to the emotional shock and grief over the death, there are often many concurrent losses. These additional losses may require many social changes. If the bereaved spouse was dependent for many things on the person who died, he'll have to learn many new skills at a time when personal resources are greatly diminished. The bereaved partner may be required to parent alone, return to work or start working, and adjust to single life. The death also may mean the loss of social contacts and activities formerly done with the spouse, which can lead to social isolation.

The elderly are vulnerable when they lose a lifetime partner, and their loneliness may be compounded by the multiple deaths of close friends. Widowed persons often feel isolated and alone, especially when family and friends return to their own lives, leaving them with no one who understands their bereavement experience. Social support, particularly with other widowed people, is very important. Encourage the person to join a bereavement group for spousal loss. Local groups often can be found through churches and non-profit organizations. Local telephone directories have a listing of available groups.

Death of a child

The loss of a parent is the loss of the past; the loss of a child is the loss of the future. Thus, it carries both physical and symbolic losses. When parents lose a child, they may lose their dreams and their identity as a parent. They typically feel a strong sense of injustice because the death of a child in current American culture is unexpected. Years after the loss, parents still experience the pain of grief from the void left by the deceased child. (See *Brooke's balloons* page 250.) They imagine what the child would be like and may grieve through the rites of passage to adulthood, such as graduation from high school.

Differences in the bereaved mother's and father's expressions of grief can lead to marital difficulties. Women are more likely to verbalize their feelings and cry, whereas men are likely to distract themselves with work. Bereaved mothers interpret their partner's lack of expression as lack of grief. You can help by bringing the normal difference among individual grief responses to the attention of families and couples. This awareness can open communication and decrease misunderstanding among surviving family members.

Sudden death If the child's death was sudden, parents may have intense feelings of guilt, real or imagined. If the child died of sudden infant death

EXPERT INSIGHTS

Brooke's balloons

I'm the father of two toddlers, so when I care for a terminally ill child, I can't help but identify with the parents. I think about them for a long time after the child's death. How does anyone deal with such a heart-breaking loss? — M. M., N.J.

Everyone copes differently, of course, but some parents find comfort in keeping the child's spirit alive for themselves and others. Your question reminds me of Brooke, who died in the pediatric unit after a courageous battle with leukemia, and her parents, who were determined to memorialize her struggle. Members of her church collected money for a commemorative plaque, which her parents wanted to place on the the floor of the room where she'd fought her disease so bravely. But hospital administrators wouldn't allow it, afraid that many similar requests might follow.

The frustrated parents called me several times. Suddenly I had an idea!

I spoke with the child's pediatrician, who was also chief of the department. He agreed that something had to be done and made a few phone calls. The next day he proudly displayed the design of a large plaque to be placed in the hospital lobby. It would list the names of any children who'd died, if their parents chose to do so. Brooke's name would be listed first, with a few words describing how the memorial came to be created. It wasn't morose or scary, and hospital administration accepted the plan.

Although Brooke's parents were pleased, they weren't completely satisfied. They still wanted her room to be special.

Suddenly I had another inspiration. Would they consider setting up a weekly delivery of nonlatex balloons to hang outside the door? They loved the idea.

"But what if a parent or child wants to know why the balloons are there?" asked the father.

"We'll just say because a very special angel wants them there to cheer up boys and girls who don't feel so good."

Brooke's father nodded, satisfied at last.

"That sounds just like something our Brooke would say."

— JOY UFEMA, RN, MS

syndrome (SIDS), the cause is unknown, and parents may struggle for years over what they could have done to prevent the death. These bereaved parents need to know why their child died. Providing information, and connecting them with others who experienced a SIDS death, is important to their recovery.

Early death Grief after a miscarriage or stillborn loss may be unrecognized and unsupported by traditional supportive structures. A conspiracy of silence follows when friends and neighbors don't talk about the child because they fear saying the wrong thing.

If the loss is a miscarriage, acknowledge it as a loss. Treat the fetus with respect. Provide details about the baby's weight, length, and hair color when possible. Move the mother to another unit or private room away from the nursery where she must hear babies crying. Make sure that all the staff knows about her loss and her grief. Over the long term, allow the bereaved parents to talk about the loss. Maintain telephone or personal contact periodically to give them the opportunity to talk if desired.

For a stillborn or newborn death, the short time for attachment with their infant leaves bereaved parents trying to accept the reality of the birth at the same time as death. Grief is facilitated by giving the parents time with the deceased child's body and with affirming the life of the child. Use the name of the child to reinforce the child's identity and existence. Parents often fear they'll forget the child. Memorializing and celebrating the life helps with this confusion. Provide concrete memories of the child such as photographs, a lock of hair, or footprints. Provide anticipatory guidance about anniversary grief responses. Encourage participation in rituals and memorials appropriate to family culture. Support having an autopsy if the cause of death is unknown. Allow and encourage the parents and siblings to talk about the death and their feelings by being an active listener. Honoring the life that was lost in a tangible memento helps the bereaved to affirm the life and grieve its loss.

Meeting others who have survived the grief that follows childhood death may give hope to newly bereaved parents and may reduce their sense of isolation. Many organizations, such as Compassionate Friends, have support groups throughout the country. For a family uninterested in a group or if no group meets in their community, try connecting them with another family who has experienced the same type of loss. Make sure to get consent from both sides before sharing the information.

Communication skills

Families that don't have good communication skills—along with empathy and respect for each other—present a liability rather than a source of support for each other after a death. Most people turn first to their family as a source of support after a family member dies. A strong family system is an important source of building strength in individual family members. The open discussion of death, in the context of cultural norms, will facilitate the expression of grief in families. In the absence of communication, the possibility of guilt, blame, and conflict increases. When a family member is dying, there are often issues that can be resolved. The ease with which the family is able to share communication about feelings is crucial to reaching closure for the survivors.

The most important intervention for bereaved families is to help the family talk openly about the death and their emotional reactions to it. Facilitate open communication by arranging the appropriate environment for sharing. In the acute care setting, find a private place for the family to gather or make sure the dying person has a private room so that multiple family members can be present. Provide guidance with more than one family member present so that information can be reinforced through discussion among those present. Asking how one family member is feeling in the presence of other family members lets them hear about emotional responses that otherwise might not have been shared. This technique can open up communication channels related to feelings of grief.

Families who don't reach out for emotional support after a death risk depleting their emotional resources through their imposed isolation. Each family will respond uniquely to the loss of a member based in part on the individual family members and on the family's culture, religion, and relationship to the community.

Nurses are with families at their most vulnerable moments, from birth to death. You can provide crucial support to individuals, provide needed referrals, and direct families to resources that will continue to help them. You have the opportunity to promote individual and family health in the face of grief and mourning.

Issues in acute care settings

18

Usually, the topic of end-of-life care brings to mind a patient dying relatively slowly, either in his home or in a hospital, residential facility, or hospice facility. The fact is, of course, that patients die in acute care settings, too, often with little time to plan what palliative workers call *a good death*. Even so, these patients and their families deserve and should receive palliative care and should be referred to palliative specialists even when there's only a short time left to live.

This is the time when patients and families most need the services of nurses and other health care professionals who understand the principles of palliative and hospice care—not just the principles of patient care but also the emotional and spiritual assistance family members desperately need. This is the time that families most need information and teaching—and a time when they're least able to listen, learn, and form realistic expectations.

When a patient is dying suddenly and unexpectedly, the family will always view the death as tragic, regardless of the patient's chronological age. Years later, they may be able to reminisce that "grandma was healthy and driving right up to end," but as their 90-year-old grandmother lies dying in an intensive care unit (ICU) after a head-on collision with a drunk driver, they're going to be angry and feel that her life was taken too soon.

When a family must abruptly confront the unexpected death of a loved one, providing care and teaching becomes more difficult because the family is overwhelmed. Indeed, when a patient is dying unexpectedly, the family may be in denial and unwilling to even discuss end-of-life care. Especially in an acute care setting, they may have to make stressful, life-changing decisions when they don't even understand the medical terminology or the stark reality they're facing. (See *One last shot*, page 254.)

EXPERT INSIGHTS

One last shot

On our oncology unit, many patients are admitted for end-of-life care. Our staff collaborates with staff from our excellent hospice program, which is affiliated with the visiting nurse association. The problem? One oncologist admits terminally ill patients who seem unaware that they're dying. Instead, they think they're in the hospital to "give it one more shot." These patients are overloaded with I.V. fluids and even tube feedings and wind up suffering needlessly. How can we help them? — G.G., Okla.

I see nothing wrong with admitting patients to the hospital for pain and symptom management. The problem here is that this oncologist sees death as a failure rather than as a natural part of life. Consequently, he and the patient never have the important conversation about alternative plans to consider "in case this cancer gets ahead of us." The patient and his family are swept along in this physician's denial and unreasonable expectations.

Palliative care specialists understand that overloading failing systems with I.V. fluids and tube feedings causes third-spacing and edema. By impairing breathing, pulmonary edema only adds to the patient's suffering.

Just as you have policies and procedures for administering chemotherapy, so too should you have guidelines regarding admission and care of terminally ill patients. If the oncologist isn't following your facility's policy, you and your nurse-manager should inform the chief of medicine and ask him to step in. If your facility doesn't have a policy for terminally ill patients, or if the policy is outdated, work through channels to develop one. Encourage participation from everyone involved in the care of these patients, including social workers and members of the ethics committee. But be especially attentive to the advice of those who "do it right" — hospice and visiting nurses and physicians who specialize in palliative care.

— *JOY UFEMA, RN, MS*

Day-to-day living, and the patient's dying, won't suddenly stop just because the family is overwhelmed and needs more time to emotionally prepare themselves. Their loved one will die regardless of the family's state of emotional preparedness. Emotions will run high, particularly when the family has little time to prepare or say goodbye. To make matters worse, in these situations, problems within the family dynamic become accentuated.

They may create an emotional minefield if the family is dysfunctional and has secrets or unresolved issues. It's the job of health care providers to make sure the patient can die peacefully and comfortably and to provide emotional support to the family during the process.

Two of the most difficult, and most important, aspects of providing care for a dying patient in an acute care setting are explaining the dying process to the patient's family and helping them through the process of weaning from a ventilator.

Explaining the dying process

Up to the point of actively dying, the patient may still be receiving aggressive treatment. Ideally, regardless of the setting, aggressive measures should be stopped when a patient is actively dying. In active dying, the patient's body is undergoing a natural shutting-down process designed to minimize pain and suffering. Continuing aggressive treatment that would help an ordinary patient recover will likely only increase the suffering of a dying patient.

The active dying phase is a protective mechanism. When you describe it to the patient's family, use terminology that will reinforce dying as a natural process that protects their loved one from pain and suffering. (See *Deciding for Nadine*, page 256.) The process entails a combination of changes in vital signs and lowered consciousness. For example, the heart rate is usually increased, often to tachycardia. Blood pressure is usually decreased, often to hypotension. Respiratory rate may be increased, decreased, or unusual, as in Cheyne-Stokes or Kussmaul's respirations. Normally, as the patient approaches death, periods of apnea will become longer and more frequent. Explain to family members that these changes are all a helpful part of the normal dying process.

Often, the patient's temperature will be elevated, especially if the patient is in fluid overload. Try to avoid the temptation to "treat" a terminal fever, either with drugs such as acetaminophen or with cold compresses or ice packs. Usually, terminal fever causes the patient no discomfort while providing a means of reducing fluid and terminal congestion, particularly as urine output decreases or stops. Explain that, unless the patient is uncomfortable, it's in the patient's best interest not to treat terminal fever.

Caring for an actively dying patient requires keeping him pain-free and comfortable. Consider pain the "fifth vital sign" and assess it at least as often as the other vital signs, more often if a patient has severe pain. In that case, check the patient's pain level every 15 minutes or less, if needed.

Other comfort steps include keeping the patient clean at all times and providing frequent mouth care. Dying patients typically breathe through their mouths, and the membranes can dry out quickly. Plain water on a

Deciding for Nadine

Our hospice service received a request to consult about a terminal patient who needed to be weaned from the ventilator. The patient was in a vegetative state after having a stroke. While the social worker spoke with the family, the hospice nurse examined the patient and reviewed the chart.

Active dying

Nadine was actively dying. Her heart rate and temperature were skyrocketing. Her blood pressure, urine output, and oxygen saturation were plummeting. Nadine was edematous and so bloated she must have been almost unrecognizable to her own family.

Trying to burn off the excess fluid, Nadine's body temperature had climbed to 104° F. Her urine output was scant, and the tubing from her Foley catheter was dotted with the rust-colored casts put out by kidneys that are shutting down. Nadine's urine was dark and thick, and a layer of the same rusty sediment rested in the bottom of the urine collection bag.

Family discussion

After her assessment, the hospice nurse joined the social worker in the family lounge to speak with the family. They were distraught. They didn't want to prematurely stop efforts to save Nadine, even though they said they understood that she was vegetative and couldn't make a meaningful recovery.

The nurse discussed the process of actively dying and explained how this related to their mother's vital signs. She reassured the family that Nadine was already dying and that, regardless of whether life support was continued or not, their mother's body was preparing itself to die. The ventilator wasn't maintaining Nadine's oxygenation, and removing it would allow the natural protective processes to occur and not cause Nadine to suffer.

Knowing that they weren't "pulling the plug too soon" relieved the family of the emotional burden they had been carrying, and they agreed to remove the ventilator. Because the patient was in fluid overload, she was given an anticholinergic drug to reduce secretions, and she was placed in an almost upright position to lessen her pulmonary congestion and risk of oropharyngeal secretions. The patient was carefully and thoroughly suctioned before extubation. The ventilator was then discontinued, and Nadine died naturally and painlessly about 36 hours later.

mouth sponge is usually the best option. If the patient's mouth is particularly encrusted, you might try alcohol-free mouth rinse. Avoid glycerin swabs because glycerin further dries the membranes. A small amount of petroleum jelly can be used to keep lips moist, but avoid excessive coating. As appropriate, teach family members to provide mouth care as a way to help their dying loved one.

Never remove an actively dying patient from his bed without a good reason. If you're practicing in an extended care facility that requires all patients not on strict bed rest to be up, dressed, and in a cardiac chair, contact hospice immediately if your patient's condition changes to active dying. The hospice physician will write appropriate orders to make sure the patient can die peacefully in bed.

Weaning from the ventilator

Often, when a patient is dying in an acute care setting, the family is emotionally overwhelmed and may be angry, guilt-wracked, or terrified. (See *Never again*, page 258.) Making the decision to remove life support may feel like more than they can bear.

However, by explaining that the patient is actively dying and that removing the ventilator and other death-delaying efforts will allow the person to die peacefully and comfortably, a huge emotional burden may be lifted from the patient's family. Use every bit of evidence at your disposal to help the family understand that their loved one is actively dying.

When the patient's status is less obvious, provide what assurance you can while clearly presenting the facts of the case. Consider, for example, a patient in multiple organ failure who is alive only because of the ventilator and drug-supported regulation of heart rate and blood pressure. Explain to the family that the drugs are masking the overt symptoms of dying and that, once the drugs are stopped, the patient will be able to use the normal protection of the dying process to have a painless natural death. Explain that you'll make sure their loved one doesn't suffer and will receive medication to supplement the body's means of protecting itself from pain.

Occasionally a patient who's alert and oriented will ask to be taken off the ventilator. (See *Lydia's cats*, page 259.) This can be very stressful for the family. Provide reassurance to both patient and family that the patient won't suffer and will be given enough medication to control discomfort.

Nothing in hospice is as emotionally charged as the family being confronted with the decision to remove their loved one from a ventilator, nor is anything so universally misunderstood. If the patient is brain dead (which, legally and practically speaking, is dead), the hospice team probably won't be involved in removing the ventilator. Instead, the family will be asked

Never again

Pinchas Weinberg had personally experienced hell on earth in a Nazi extermination camp during World War II. After being liberated, he left Europe for a new life in America.

Pinchas wasn't well even before the stroke that brought him to the intensive care unit. He had stage IV cancer and multiple chronic health problems. After the massive stroke, it was clear that Pinchas would never recover. The question was how best to treat a dying holocaust survivor.

Palliative care consult

To start, hospice was called in to do a palliative care consult so the family could discuss having Pinchas admitted as an inpatient hospice patient. Because he had starved almost to death in the extermination camp, his family wanted everything done to make sure that Pinchas would be comfortable and never starve again. In their minds, withholding food and fluids wasn't an acceptable option.

Because this patient's care was such an emotionally charged issue for the Weinberg family, an orthodox rabbi who also was an experienced hospice chaplain was brought in to consult on the case.

Because no one could be fully certain that Pinchas would die, the family chose not to adopt hospice right away, and they chose to provide him with nutrition and fluids. However, to avoid causing Pinchas additional pain from an unnecessary procedure, the family and care team decided that he could be fed and hydrated through a nasogastric tube rather than placing a gastrostomy tube in him.

A natural death

Pinchas continued to decline despite everything being done, and the care team began teaching the family about the protective mechanism of a natural death. They learned that, rather than causing suffering, dehydration can actually help dying patients achieve a painless death. The family began to understand that feeding and hydration would only make Pinchas less comfortable.

The rabbi again spoke with the family and discussed a passage from the Talmud that addresses the special protection afforded to the dying under Jewish law. When a person is obviously actively dying, Jewish law precludes any interference that would prolong the act of dying and thereby cause more suffering.

Pinchas was put on a continuous morphine drip, and the family no longer demanded additional hydration. Pinchas died peacefully with his family at his side. Because of the support of hospice and a hospice rabbi in addressing the special needs of this family, Pinchas was spared additional suffering from interventions that wouldn't have helped him.

Lydia's cats

Lydia Johnson and her unmarried, middle-aged daughter were breeders of champion Siamese cats. Confined to her bed in the intensive care unit (ICU) of a small community hospital, Lydia was tortured by being separated from her cats. Lydia's daughter visited at least twice a day and often brought new photographs of the cats for her mother to see. A plush toy cat shared Lydia's bed.

Saying good-bye
Lydia knew she was dying and she didn't wish to be maintained on the ventilator. But she also wanted to see her cats and say good-bye. Because the ICU wasn't conducive to her request, Lydia was moved to the floor where hospice patients normally stayed. Once Lydia was settled in her private room, her daughter went home to get the cats. She received more than a few curious looks as she entered the hospital elevator with three carriers stacked on a wheeled cart.

Lydia was delighted to see her beloved friends. The nurses told Lydia to take as long as she wanted and to signal when she grew too tired. Then they closed the door to her room, the cats climbed onto the bed, and Lydia, her daughter, and the cats were given some privacy to say good-bye. When Lydia tired, the cats went back into their carriers and Lydia dozed while her daughter took the cats home.

Removing the ventilator
When her daughter returned, Lydia signaled that she was ready. The two women were given a few extra minutes alone. Lydia was given medication in her I.V. tubing to decrease discomfort and respiratory secretions on extubation, and she drifted into a light sleep. After the medication took effect, the respiratory therapist and hospice nurse were ready to shut off the vent and extubate Lydia. Her daughter was asked to step out, only for a moment, while the tube was removed.

Lydia's daughter returned to the room and gently held her mother's hand as Lydia's breathing became slower and shallower. Off the ventilator, her oxygen levels dropped quickly and she slipped deeper into unconsciousness. She breathed on her own for a few minutes, then died peacefully.

about organ donation by a special team of practitioners experienced in organ donation. If the family agrees, the patient will be taken to an operating room for organ harvesting.

Asking a family about organ donation is a difficult and delicate matter. The family deserves privacy, and this subject shouldn't be discussed in a public area or with other people present. The family should be taken to a private room and given time alone to discuss the option. Regardless of your personal feelings on the subject, you must respect the wishes of the family. Be compassionate, and support and respect their decision, whatever it is.

Weaning procedures

For a dying patient, a terminal wean from a ventilator isn't euthanasia. The patient isn't given lethal amounts of drugs. If present, paralytic drugs are discontinued and the patient is given drugs to prevent the sensation of air hunger if oxygen levels fall. If the patient will be extubated, he usually receives additional medication to promote relaxation before removal of the endotracheal tube. The patient then has the opportunity to live or die naturally.

There are three main ways to withdraw ventilator support. The most common procedure is to extubate the patient and turn off the ventilator. The second is not to extubate the patient but to substitute a T-bar for the ventilator. This is the most common procedure for patients who have a tracheostomy. The third is to use a stepped procedure to withdraw support but not extubate, in part to avoid the almost inevitable congestion caused by removal of the endotracheal tube, which allows fluid and saliva into the patient's airway. The inflated cuff of the endotracheal tube provides a mechanical barrier to prevent this fluid from entering the airway.

The decision of when or if the patient should be extubated should be based on patient comfort and the patient's (or family's) preference, religious beliefs, and state laws. For example, orthodox Jewish law doesn't allow anything to be removed from a body after death. If a patient dies with an endotracheal tube or other tubes in place, he'll be buried with them in place. Some patients prefer to die without the encumbrance of the endotracheal tube and other tubes, such as a Foley catheter. Keep in mind that, if the patient will have an autopsy, you may not be permitted to remove anything from the patient after he dies.

Although this may seem counterintuitive, most patients don't benefit from 100% oxygen after extubation. If given humidified room air or 2 L/ minute of oxygen via nasal cannula, their oxygen saturations drop faster and they go to sleep rather than developing agitation as their oxygen levels fall. This is the theory behind several versions of stepped withdrawal of ventilator support; by ventilating the patient with progressively less oxygen or with room air and reducing either the rate or volume, the patient quickly becomes hypoxic and hypercarbic. Increased carbon dioxide levels quickly lead to loss of consciousness, and the patient can die peacefully.

Expert assistance

A poorly managed terminal wean can be difficult for the patient and difficult for the patient's family to watch. However, even when managed perfectly, termination of a patient's ventilator support can be unnerving.

Occasionally, a phenomenon called the Lazarus sign occurs, probably trig-gered by hypoxia, in which certain spinal motor neurons fire and a brain-dead patient may move or even sit up. If this occurs in the presence of the family, it may be difficult to convince them that the patient is actually dead.

The vast majority of patients who are terminally weaned are actively dy-ing. By removing the ventilator, the patient is allowed to go through the protective process that a natural death affords to prevent suffering. Even though a prescribed terminal wean usually ends in death, patients do occa-sionally recover spontaneously. (See *Patient's choice*, pages 262 and 263.) A very small number end up going home, perhaps to have hospice care at home.

If you're inexperienced at terminating ventilator support, don't do it un-til you've seen it done properly several times. Also, don't let yourself be talked into undermedicating a patient by an attending physician unfamiliar with the protocols. If you're ever asked to deviate from the established pro-tocol by undermedicating a patient, ask your medical director to discuss it with the attending physician. The hospice service may decline to wean the patient, and the medical director may suggest that the attending physician do it personally if he chooses to follow another process that may risk caus-ing the patient to suffer.

Taking time

Most patients on ventilators are in the ICU. Although the ICU is a wonder-ful place to recover, it can be a bad place to die. All the invasive, aggressive measures used to preserve life in the ICU tend to result in a painful and symptomatic death. The process of actively dying is a protective mecha-nism that lowers consciousness, and ICU protocols intervene at each step to try to reverse this natural process.

Although many ICU nurses are well qualified to wean a patient from a ventilator, the length of unbroken time needed to do it properly may not be available to them because of the needs of other patients in the ICU. Most hospices are more than willing to come into acute care facilities to do the weaning and free up the ICU staff to save other patients' lives. Protocols in place at particular institutions may dictate the choices of medications and other elements of the patient's terminal weaning.

Terminal weaning takes time. There's no way to skip steps or speed up the process. Medications may have to be ordered from the hospital pharma-cy, and they'll need time to be delivered. Paralytic drugs may need time to wear off before the terminal wean can continue. Although policy usually re-quires that the patient be monitored at the nursing station until death, all of the alarms and monitor screens in the patient's room or cubicle need to be disabled before the patient is removed from life support. Unless the pa-tient expires soon after the ventilator is disconnected, the patient will have

Patient's choice

Lying in the intensive care unit (ICU) of a massive medical complex, Marie Fitzpatrick was clearly dying. She was deep blue from cyanosis. She was also alert, oriented, and bucking her ventilator. She was acutely uncomfortable and wanted to be extubated.

A clear gesture

Marie's physician preferred to sedate her and administer paralytic drugs so Marie wouldn't fight the ventilator that was keeping her alive. Marie shook her head adamantly in refusal. She gestured to remove the tube in her throat. The physician looked her squarely in the eye and asked if she understood that she would die when the tube was removed. Marie nodded that she understood.

To be absolutely clear, he rephrased the question, "Marie, do you want me to take the tube out, knowing that you will die off the ventilator?" Marie again nodded and gestured to extubate her. The physician told her he would call hospice and they would perform the procedure. Marie nodded and settled back into her bed.

Seven of Marie's eight adult children crowded around her ICU bed; the missing son was overseas, trying to get a flight back. The emotional state of this family ranged from distraught to hysterical. The patient was suffering and impatient. She wanted to proceed with the terminal wean. Marie's children cried, cajoled, begged, and pleaded with their mother to change her mind.

Calming reassurance

The hospice nurse arrived to explain the procedure to the family and get the paperwork signed for the procedure. Marie's children said they feared that their mother would be "given a shot and put down like a dog." The hospice nurse reassured them several times that their mother would be given only enough medication to make her comfortable. Knowing that this family was Roman Catholic and had a strong faith, she added that what happened afterward was up to Marie and to God.

Marie was put on a low-dose morphine drip. The nurse explained several times that morphine was a cardiac drug that would open the blood vessels around Marie's heart, give her heart more oxygen, and make her feel much less short of breath. Marie was also given an I.V. push of medication to prepare her for the extubation.

The extubation and ventilator removal went well, and the morphine and other drugs made Marie comfortable enough to doze. The morphine had allowed Marie to "pink up" and she looked peaceful and comfortable. The physician wrote an order to continue the low-dose infusion, and Marie was moved to the hospice wing to die.

Patient's choice *(continued)*

When the hospice nurse arrived at Marie's room the next morning, Marie was sitting up in bed and had eaten everything on her breakfast tray. She clearly was not dying at that moment and told the nurse that she was eager to regain her strength. The nurse explained that she could revoke the hospice benefit if she wished and could return if she got sicker. Marie elected to revoke hospice and go home, knowing that if she ever needed it, hospice was still available.

---

to be carefully monitored for signs of respiratory distress for 60 to 90 minutes or more.

Ideally, protocols for terminating ventilator support should be written or updated to accommodate patient (or family) preference and prevent patient suffering. The protocols need to accommodate the range of patients undergoing the procedure, from those who are brain dead to those who are alert and oriented. Decisions about how ventilator support should be removed should be based on sound evidence-based practice, not on an arbitrary protocol.

Family challenges

The timing of a person's death depends on several factors, including the person's will to live, his overall state of physical health, and his terminal diagnosis. Dying young people are at a disadvantage because their strong healthy hearts want to keep beating, and these patients usually are highly motivated to live. This combination can lead to physical, emotional, and spiritual suffering. Patients continue to fight until they reach their own personal limit. When their quality of life drops, and that limit is reached, they give up and usually die very quickly.

Dying patients sometimes live much longer than their prognosis because they're committed to living long enough to do a particular thing. (See *Easter blessing,* pages 264 and 265.) The patient may focus on an upcoming holiday, a planned celebration, or some other milestone, with a single-minded purpose to live long enough to be there for it.

For some families, hospice will provide a supportive environment that allows the experience of a loved one's death to be transformational and a time of great emotional and spiritual growth. For other families it will take intense intervention on the part of social work and spiritual care just to

Easter blessing

Gizela Sobitski was a proud Polish-American lady who, years earlier, had been diagnosed with kidney cancer and breast cancer. Twice she had survived and been deemed cancer-free. "Zel" was an active senior citizen, a widow who bowled and played pinochle regularly with her ladies' club. Having beaten cancer twice, Zel felt she was indestructible.

The day Zel woke up in pain and severe respiratory distress, she immediately called her son, an intensive care unit (ICU) nurse. When he heard his mother gasping, he told her to hang up and call 911; he'd meet her at the emergency room.

End-stage status

An X-ray immediately found Zel's problem. A huge tumor enveloped her heart and penetrated far into her left lung, which had collapsed. Although Zel's lung reinflated, at least temporarily, she clearly had reached end-stage status. Zel's other sons arrived, and Zel had a long cry with her children before being discharged to receive home hospice care.

Because, secretly, no one believed that she'd live until Easter, the family planned a special party, a huge Polish-style feast, for the day before Ash Wednesday. They'd hold their big Easter party 40 days early so Zel could have a final celebration with her family. They served nearly all the traditional Easter foods so that Zel could have a celebration much like Easter itself.

A real celebration

As soon as the pretend Easter celebration was finished, Zel decided she wanted a real celebration. She invited cousins from Poland and special-ordered Polish delicacies. The idea was preposterous. To plan a party 40 days in the future was entirely unrealistic.

Day by day, Zel declined. Week by week, her condition went from bad to worse. Zel's left lung slowly deflated and was moving no air. Her right lung also wasn't fully functional. Rather than give up or cancel the party, Zel spent about 3 weeks in bed lying on her left side. By lying on the deflated lung, she could hyperexpand the functional portion of the right lung and actually breathe.

At first, Zel's son—the ICU nurse—tried to turn his mother, concerned about skin breakdown. But after turning her a few times and watching his mother grow deep blue, he decided to leave her alone. Zel did get some rather extensive skin breakdown on her left side, but she was adamant about her Easter party.

> **Easter blessing** *(continued)*
>
> Amazingly enough, Zel actually improved just before Easter. Her left lung partly reinflated, and she could move air in the top of the upper lobe. The woman who had turned deep blue days before was able to eat Easter dinner with her family, including her cousins from Poland. They said it was the best Easter the family ever had.
>
> Zel had a wonderful time, surrounded by her family. She stayed up with the family until her grandchildren tired. But eventually Zel admitted that she was exhausted and asked for help in getting to bed. She spent the next day in bed, too tired to get up. The following day, she went into a coma. Two days later, she died.

keep their powder keg of emotions from becoming explosive. Some families will find the stress of the situation overwhelming and will be torn apart by the impending death. Other families will rise to the occasion, overcome their differences, achieve reconciliation, and strengthen their family's bond.

Expect the family of a dying patient to have complicated problems just like most every other family. An alcoholic caregiver won't start detoxification and rehabilitation in the midst of his loved one's dying process. The death of a loved one won't magically eliminate problems in a dysfunctional family and may worsen them. The goal is to provide enough support to help the family through the crisis; how they choose to deal with their particular family issues is up to them, although the hospice team may be able to make useful referrals or suggestions for ongoing care.

Palliative care is about allowing death to be dignified and comfortable by alleviating suffering and allowing the body to follow its natural protective course. Death isn't the enemy; if there's an enemy, it's suffering.

PART FOUR

Supporting the staff

19 Documenting care

Proper nursing documentation provides a record of your nursing care. Detailed standards have been developed by the Joint Commission on Accreditation of Healthcare Organizations (JCAHO) to guide the documentation of a patient's care up to and after death. These standards emphasize the integration of services from a variety of providers. They include assessment and care of patients, leadership, management of human resources, and ongoing data collection.

Clearly, documentation is as important for a dying patient as it is for any other patient. In the area of end-of-life care, certain issues in documentation deserve special mention. These include understanding the type of documentation you'll be using and documenting pain control, advance directives, Medicare requirements, organ donation, and documentation after death.

Documenting pain control

Documentation of pain control is essential as the patient progresses through the dying process. When charting pain levels and characteristics of discomfort, document the location of the pain and whether it's internal, external, localized, or diffuse. Using the patient's own words, describe his pain, emphasizing how long the pain lasts, how often it occurs, as well as his ranking of the pain using a numerical, visual, or verbal scale.

Also describe the patient's behaviors associated with the pain, and record changes in blood pressure, dilated pupils, shortness of breath, elevated heart rate, and diaphoresis. Chart positions and measures that relieve or worsen

Patient-controlled analgesia: Flowsheet documentation

Although each facility will vary slightly in its requirements, certain elements are typically included in documenting patient-controlled analgesia (PCA) on a flowsheet:

- Type of drug used, including mixture amounts
- Time of cartridge insertion
- PCA settings, including lockout interval
- Dose volume
- Continuous settings
- 4-hour limit
- Vital signs
- Rating of level of sedation
- Rating of level of pain
- Additional doses given
- Total milliliters of analgesic given
- Total milliliters remaining in medication cartridge

the pain. A pain flowsheet can be invaluable in documenting pain occurrence and describing its characteristics. It can be particularly beneficial for families involved in caring for a loved one at home because they may be overwhelmed by a lengthy, detailed questionnaire. A pain flowsheet should include at least the following five categories:

- date and time of every occurrence of pain
- patient rating of pain from 0 to 10 when pain occurs
- patient behaviors with each occurrence of pain
- patient rating of pain from 0 to 10 after intervention to relieve pain
- description of drugs given or other measures taken for pain relief.

As the patient continues to move through the dying process, he may use patient-controlled analgesia. This lets the patient self-administer boluses of an opioid analgesic intravenously, subcutaneously, or epidurally within prescribed limits. Patient-controlled analgesia increases the patient's sense of control, reduces his anxiety, reduces the amount of analgesic used, and increases pain control. This type of pain relief is particularly effective when used with terminal cancer patients.

When documenting the use of patient-controlled analgesia with a dying patient, make sure to include the name of the opioid used, the lockout interval, the maintenance dose used, the amount of drug the patient receives when he activates the device, and the amount of opioid used during your shift. Record the patient's assessment of pain relief, patient teaching performed, vital signs, and level of consciousness, as well as observations of the insertion site. (See *Patient-controlled analgesia: Flowsheet documentation.*)

Advance directives

An advance directive is a legal document executed by the patient while he is of sound mind that dictates his wishes should he become incapacitated and unable to make decisions. Under ideal circumstances, the patient has discussed his wishes with his family members and they agree to his desired outcomes. However, there may be situations in which family members contest the patient's wishes for the advance directive. The legality of the situation dictates that the living will be upheld. The family's rights will be superseded by the living will.

Should such contention occur, notify the physician, the nursing supervisor, and the facility's risk manager. Document conversations held with the family members, quoting their exact words. Record an assessment of the family dynamics. Document the name and department of all personnel notified. Consider making a referral to the facility's ethics committee or patient advocate, and document all referrals made.

 ALERT If the patient wishes not to be resuscitated, inform the practitioner and request that a signed do-not-resuscitate (DNR) order be placed in his chart.

Even if a patient has an advance directive, it should be reviewed yearly and updated as needed. The advance directive will only become effective if the conditions under which the patient has defined the document to be activated have occurred. The advance directive may be revoked by the patient at any time. If the patient decides to revoke his advance directive, place a copy of his written revocation in the medical record, or sign and date a statement in the patient's own words explaining that the patient made the request orally. Include names of witnesses who heard the patient revoke his advance directive. Record that the physician, risk manager, and nursing supervisor were notified of the revocation.

Interdisciplinary team

The emphasis of hospice and palliative care is on the benefits of all disciplines working together to assist the patient and family to achieve their goals. Documentation of interactions of interdisciplinary team members is essential. In hospitals, the progress note is typically used by all disciplines and can serve this function. In extended care facilities, home care, and inpatient hospice settings, it may be helpful to have a form dedicated to this function. The form should identify which problem was discussed, based on the care plan established for that patient. The specific people involved should also be identified; include the patient or family when appropriate.

Interdisciplinary team meeting record

No.	Problem	Notes	Members present
1.	Bladder: dysuria, frequency, nocturia, incontinence, retention		❑ Chaplain
2.	Body fluids: dehydration, ascites, edema		❑ Dietary
3.	Bowel: constipation, impaction, incontinence, diarrhea		❑ Home health aide
4.	Cognitive alteration		❑ Hospice coordinator
5.	Communication alteration		❑ Hospice director
6.	Confusion or disorientation		❑ Hospice secretary
7.	Discomfort or pain		❑ Nurse
8.	Infection, inflammation, and immune system		❑ Occupational therapy
9.	Medications		❑ Pharmacy
10.	Nutrition: obesity, anorexia, nausea, decreased intake, vomiting, dysphagia		❑ Physical therapy
11.	Respiratory dysfunction: dyspnea, cough, orthopnea		❑ Physician
12.	Rest and sleep		❑ Social services
13.	Sensory alteration		❑ Speech therapy
14.	Skin impairments: wounds, lesions, decubiti		❑ Volunteer
			❑ Volunteer coordinator
			❑ Other

The note should include the interventions agreed upon, which team members will carry them out, and an expected timeline for re-evaluation. (See *Interdisciplinary team meeting record*.)

Medicare measures

Documentation is an integral part of the process of providing hospice care to a patient under the Medicare hospice benefit. Hospice care specifically refers to services provided for a terminally ill patient who has been judged by two physicians as having a life expectancy of 6 months or less.

To access Medicare's hospice benefits, when hospice care is desired, the patient must file an election statement with a Medicare-certified hospice. When hospice care is elected by the patient, he waives all rights to Medicare payments for treatments related to the terminal illness and instead receives hospice care for the terminal illness. However, if the patient also needs care for conditions unrelated to his terminal illness, he can receive hospice as well as Medicare-reimbursed health benefits.

Hospice in nursing homes

Hospice care is also being used to provide skills and services in nursing homes. The National Hospice Organization has published guidelines to help determine the appropriateness of a chronically ill patient to receive hospice care. Documentation is particularly important in this instance because the guidelines require frequent reevaluation of the patient's condition to monitor disease progression. Based on the guidelines, an eligible patient would be unable to bathe properly, have urinary and fecal incontinence, be unable to ambulate without assistance, be unable to dress without assistance, and be unable to speak or communicate meaningfully.

Once a nursing home resident is identified as having a limited life expectancy, it's important to recognize that the Medicare hospice benefit can assist in providing palliative management of the dying patient's symptoms, paying particular attention to the patient's increased daily needs and supplying bereavement services. (See *Services covered by the Medicare hospice benefit.*)

When a nursing home resident is referred for care under the Medicare hospice benefit, the hospice assumes responsibility for management of the interdisciplinary services that will supplement the usual care provided by nursing home staff. The process of delivering end-of-life care will continue within the dual regulations of the nursing home and the hospice. In terms of documentation, the care plan must reflect the hospice philosophy and must be based on an assessment of the patient's needs and specific living arrangement in the nursing home. The plan of care must document the resident's current medical, physical, psychosocial, and spiritual needs. Since the care plan will be coordinated between the nursing home and hospice, it must also designate which care and services the nursing home will consistently provide.

During the provision of hospice services in a nursing home setting, the attending physician remains in charge and works cooperatively with the interdisciplinary team. The physician will usually order the personalized medical care, including pain control and relief of common symptoms of the dying process, such as dyspnea.

Services covered by the Medicare hospice benefit

- Hospice nursing care under the supervision of a registered nurse who usually has special training and expertise in end-of-life care (The hospice nurse will visit the patient as needed and is on call along with other hospice nurses 24 hours a day, 7 days a week to provide support to the nursing home staff, patient, and family members.)
- Medical social services and counseling provided by a social worker
- Consultation and oversight provided by hospice medical director
- Bereavement counseling, including adjustment-to-death support for the patient's family, and bereavement services for 1 year after the patient's death
- Compassionate listening and companionship for the patient and family from trained hospice volunteers
- Physical, occupational, speech therapy, and dietary services as needed to improve quality of life and safety
- Home health aide services
- Drugs and medical supplies provided by the hospice as needed for palliation and management of the terminal illness and related conditions (The patient is responsible for a 5% drug copayment, not to exceed $5 per drug.)
- Pastoral care assessment and services, if desired

In the nursing home setting, some drugs essential for comprehensive hospice care are typically controlled under regulations set by the Omnibus Reconciliation Act. However, if you document their use appropriately in the patient's chart and care plan, the drugs can be used.

Home care without hospice

If a patient is seriously ill and is receiving home health services, he may ultimately die at home without the benefit of hospice if the physician has never judged him to be terminally ill or he has elected to not use the Medicare hospice benefit for his care. You must know the correct documentation to use in order to complete all required paperwork according to Medicare regulations. All Medicare-certified home health agencies are required to complete a comprehensive assessment of home health patients using a standardized data set called the Outcome and Assessment Information Set (OASIS). OASIS allows you to collect data to measure changes in a patient's health status over time. OASIS data will typically need to be collected when a patient is enrolled into home care, at the 60-day recertification point, and when he is discharged. Remember that a patient's death will still warrant discharge information.

Use of OASIS can cost a home health agency thousands of dollars if you don't complete all areas of documentation. The OASIS material uses a point system for certain questions, and these points determine the reimbursement to be received by the agency. For example, if a patient has multiple areas of skin breakdown, each area must be documented appropriately or the home health agency may not receive adequate reimbursement for the care and supplies delivered.

Another essential piece of documentation in home health nursing is the comprehensive plan of care. The care plan should be developed with the patient and his caregivers and should reflect adjustment of interventions, patient goals, and teaching accordingly. (See *Home health care plan.*) If the patient's condition is deteriorating and it appears that death may be imminent, particularly if he has a do-not-resuscitate order, the plan of care should reflect these changes in condition. If the patient dies unexpectedly, the home care plan can be used as legal evidence because it provides the most direct legal evidence of nursing judgment. If a particular care plan is outlined and you deviate from it without documenting a good reason for doing so, the court may decide that you've strayed from a reasonable standard of care. The care plan must be updated routinely so it accurately reflects clinical judgment regarding the care needed for the patient, particularly if he is terminally ill. As the patient's condition changes, document that the changes were reported to the physician. This will ensure reimbursement by Medicare and other insurers with similar policies such as Medicaid.

When the patient dies, a discharge summary must be completed for the case to be closed and for reimbursers to be notified that services have been terminated. Although forms vary from agency to agency, certain topics are essential for completion of a discharge summary. Be sure to include physician and family notification of the patient's death, a description of the patient's physical and emotional condition when death occurred, and support systems and referrals for bereavement care made.

Organ donation documentation

Part of the documentation required when a patient dies is related to organ donation. A federal requirement enacted in 1998 requires facilities to report deaths to the regional organ procurement organization. Enacted so that no potential donor would be missed, the regulation ensures that the family of every potential donor will understand the option to donate. Collection of most organs, particularly the heart, liver, kidney, and pancreas, requires

Home health care plan

A comprehensive home health care plan includes at least the following information:
- demographic information and diagnoses
- documentation that the patient is homebound, a requirement for Medicare home health reimbursement
- prognosis
- measures to ensure the patient's safety
- list of resources the patient will need
- list of activities that the patient can perform
- discharge plans
- description of primary caregiver, relationship to patient, whether she lives with the patient, her age and physical ability, and her willingness to help the patient
- information about drugs the patient is taking
- nutritional requirements
- mental status
- rehabilitation potential, including functional limitations
- orders for physical or speech therapy
- treatments needed (amount, frequency, and duration)
- use of durable medical equipment and supplies
- patient's goals
- emotional states and attitudes of patient, family, and caregiver
- information about the home environment and assistance the family will need to give care in a safe environment
- ways to encourage the patient to utilize his support systems (including physician, pharmacist, and members of the health care team) and resources (medical equipment, coping behaviors, and financial planning).

that the patient be pronounced brain dead and kept physically alive until organ harvest occurs. Tissue such as eyes, skin, bone, and heart valves may be taken after death. Each facility must have a policy for identifying and reporting a potential organ donor. The local or regional organ procurement organization must be contacted when a potential donor is identified.

Asking the family

Usually, a specially trained person from the facility along with someone from the regional organ procurement organization will speak with the family regarding organ donation. The organ procurement organization will coordinate the donation process after a family consents to donation.

The first step in making a referral to the organ procurement organization is to ensure that the medical chart is available so the patient's diagnosis and background can be reviewed. Information that's usually needed includes:

■ patient's name, age, sex, race, medical and social history, current diagnoses, nursing unit where patient died, and date and time of death

■ information adequate to determine whether any conditions could prevent donation, such as hospital course of treatment, results of blood culture, and medications received by the patient

■ name and telephone number of patient's next of kin.

It's the responsibility of the organ procurement organization to request organ and tissue donation from the family. Organ donation occurs most often when a patient is declared brain dead, although tissue donation is an option for patients who experience cardiac death or brain death. (See *Criteria for organ and tissue donation.*)

Defining death

Death is considered imminent when the patient is ventilator-maintained and appears to have experienced an irreversible loss of brain function. When a state of imminent death is present, the organ procurement organization should be notified immediately and certainly must be notified before removing the patient from the ventilator. Early referrals to the organ procurement organization are essential because the patient's family must be given adequate time to be educated about donation, to discuss options, and to make an informed decision while the patient's stability is being maintained so that donation remains medically possible if the family gives consent.

Usually, to be an organ donor, the patient must have been declared brain dead and be maintained on a ventilator. Brain death may occur after the patient experiences head trauma, anoxic injuries, cerebral bleeding, or a brain tumor. To help physicians determine brain death, an ad hoc committee at Harvard Medical School published a report in 1968 that established specific criteria for determination of brain death, including:

■ failure to respond to the most painful environmental stimuli

■ absence of spontaneous respiratory or muscular movement

■ absence of reflexes

■ flat electroencephalogram.

The committee recommended that all tests be repeated after 24 hours and that hypothermia and central nervous system depressants be eliminated. Ultimately, the Uniform Determination of Death Act was de-

Criteria for organ and tissue donation

Brain death
■ The patient is maintained on a ventilator with his heart beating.
■ The patient is a viable candidate for organ and tissue donation.
■ Tissue recovery follows organ procurement.

Cardiac death
■ The patient has no cardiac or respiratory activity.
■ The patient is a candidate for tissue donation unless the hospital has adopted a policy against donation after cardiac death.
■ The body must be kept cool before tissue recovery.
■ Recovery of tissues must occur within 24 hours of death.

veloped, which defines brain death as the cessation of all measurable functions or activity in every area of the brain, including the brain stem. This definition excludes comatose patients as well as those who exist in a persistent vegetative state.

The physician's clinical examination will include an evaluation of overall level of responsiveness, brain-stem reflexes, and apnea testing. Nurse's notes for a patient undergoing testing for brain death should include:
■ date and time of each test
■ name of the test
■ name of person performing the test
■ response of the patient to the test
■ actions taken in response to the patient, such as the course of action if an arrhythmia develops
■ time and names of personnel notified of results of tests
■ support provided to family members if present.

Tissue and eye donation could occur after either brain death or cardiac death because patients don't need to be maintained on ventilators for tissue or eye donation to take place. This increases the opportunities for patients to become tissue donors after death. For organ donation to occur after cardiac death:
■ a patient must have experienced devastating and unrecoverable brain damage leading to ventilator dependency
■ the family has opted to withdraw mechanical ventilation
■ death from cardiac and respiratory arrest will occur within 1 hour after withdrawal of mechanical support.

As part of documentation required during the organ donation process, record the date and time that the patient was pronounced brain dead and the physician's discussions with the family regarding prognosis. If the patient's driver's license or other documents indicate his wish to become a donor, place copies in the medical record and document their placement. The nurse who contacted the regional organ procurement organization must document the conversation, including the date and time it occurred, the name of the person spoken to, and all instructions received. Regarding discussions with the family about organ donation, document who was present, information provided to the family and by whom, and their response. Record all nursing care of the donor until the time that he is transported to the operating room for the procurement procedure to begin. Finally, chart all teaching, explanations, and emotional support given to the family.

Documentation after death

The death of a long-term patient can be traumatic not only for family members but for the nurses who have provided daily care and have become part of his support system during the dying process. However, part of remaining an advocate for a patient who has died, as well as for his family, is continued accurate documentation. This ensures that his remains are treated with dignity and that his postmortem wishes are carried out appropriately.

After a patient dies, postmortem care will include preparing his body for family viewing, comforting family members as they grieve, providing them with privacy, arranging for family members to sign a permit allowing the body to be transported to a funeral home of their choice, and determining the disposition of the patient's belongings. In some states, registered nurses are also permitted to initiate the death certificate for patients documented to be receiving only palliative care.

Preparing for autopsy

Postmortem care usually will begin after a physician certifies the patient's body and signs the death certificate. However, if an autopsy is expected, postmortem care may be postponed until after the autopsy is finished.

Although regulations may vary from state to state, consent for a postmortem examination of a body by a physician may be given by a parent, spouse, child, guardian, or next of kin of the deceased person. Consent may be in the form of a written document, a telegram, or a phone conversation. The patient will be transferred from the nursing unit to the morgue to await autopsy. It's vital that you make sure the patient has proper identification, either as a toe tag or a wrist band, or the autopsy won't be performed.

The autopsy also won't be performed unless the body arrives in the morgue with the chart and permission form. The physician who completes the autopsy usually must file a report with the office designated by the autopsy order by the 30th day after the autopsy date unless the physician certifies when the autopsy report is filed that a required test couldn't be completed within the 30-day time limit.

Once it's determined that consent for an autopsy will be needed, document the time and date of the patient's death and the name of the physician (or nurse, in some states) who pronounced death. If resuscitation took place, indicate the time it started and ended, referring to the code sheet that will be in the patient's medical record. State if the case is being referred to the medical examiner. If it becomes your responsibility to obtain a death certificate for a deceased patient, a copy may be obtained for a fee from each state's Bureau of Vital Statistics, which usually is associated with the state's Public Health Department.

Postmortem care

Describe all postmortem care provided, noting removal of medical equipment such as feeding tubes and I.V. lines. List all belongings and valuables and the name of the family member who took them and signed the personal effects list. Record any belongings remaining with the patient—for example, if dentures remained in the patient's mouth or if family asked for the wedding ring to remain on the patient's finger. Document the disposition of the patient's body and the name, telephone number, and address of the receiving funeral home. List names of family members who were present at the time of death. If for cultural or religious reasons the family performed the personal cleansing of the body, document that as well. If family members were not in attendance, provide the name of the family member who was notified. Note all care, emotional support, and education provided to the family.

Regardless of the interventions performed and their method of implementation, documenting all actions provided to ensure the comfort of the dying patient and the emotional care of his family remains an essential part of the process of end-of-life care. Such documentation provides tangible evidence of the palliative care team's commitment to providing physical and emotional care and comfort to the dying patient.

20 | Living with dying

Nurses enter into hospice and palliative care practice for our own special and individual reasons. Some of us have experienced our own losses and hope to make the transition to death a healing experience for others. Some of us have recognized the truth of our own mortality—understanding that, as humans, our fate (and perhaps our gift) is knowing that we will someday die. Some of us come to work with dying people to learn and to ease the passage in whatever ways we can, by being midwives to the dying.

Our reasons for entering this type of nursing practice vary, and the day-to-day experience of working with dying people will affect each of us differently. Despite our differences, however, we share some commonalities. These include the importance of reflection, the need to pull from abundance in providing care, the sometimes difficult task of maintaining compassion for others and ourselves, and the need to maintain balance in our lives.

We also need expertise in dealing with difficult family dynamics and responding to family situations that create discomfort and dissent. Finally, we need ways to obtain support through our systems, our colleagues, and our own attention to self-care—a required quality that allows us to stay grounded in the midst of suffering.

A view of death

Western civilization as we know it is largely a death-denying culture. We've changed death from a natural personal and social event to a technology-driven medical event. Palliative care principles are designed to ease suffering at least in part by reframing death as a natural part of life.

The dying process has been compared to the birthing process, and the analogy is useful. Both birthing and dying are natural parts of life that involve physical, psychological, and spiritual dimensions. There's nothing

---

Strategies for rehumanizing death

■ Reintroduce a peaceful sense of harmony between dying people and the process of dying.
■ Provide the support of community participation in dying rituals.
■ Support the harmonious acceptance of death as ordinary and natural, not a social evil.
■ Emphasize the comforting roles of fellowship, ritual, and ceremony.
■ Facilitate, even mandate, the notion that dying should be a culturally shared community experience.
■ Culturally legitimize the pain and suffering that often accompanies dying.
■ Provide a common base of participation and sense of belonging; attach the dying person to the community of living.

---

clean or easy about either one. And these natural processes have been going on as long as life has existed; medicalization is but a recent trend.

The problem with medicalization is that it may dehumanize life experiences. There are several strategies that can be used to transform the medicalized frame in which our culture experiences death. (See *Strategies for rehumanizing death.*)

Nurses working in the field of palliative care are, of course, committed to many of these strategies. However, dissonance may arise when the cultural view of death as a negative experience collides with the palliative care view that death is a natural part of life. This can lead to isolation. Palliative care nurses may not be able to speak openly about their work in social situations because people prefer not to think about death. There's little cultural space for discussing the profoundly life-altering experiences witnessed during end-of-life care.

All the more important, then, are the skills and characteristics you'll need to cultivate to work successfully with dying patients. These include understanding how to monitor your own strengths and limitations, how to deal in a healthy way with difficult patient and family dynamics, and how to work successfully within institutional influences.

Know thyself

When working in an emotionally powerful profession such as palliative care nursing, it's essential to cultivate self-awareness. Working with dying people is a constant reminder of our human vulnerability. The term vulnerable comes from the Latin word *vulnare*, which means *capable of being*

Validating affect and enhancing insight

Validating affect
- Supports the other by listening and acknowledging
- Allows the recipient to feel heard and understood
- Can be provided by an individual or a group

Enhancing insight
- Helps the other to work through feelings
- Encourages the other to broaden perspectives
- Can be provided by an individual or a group

---

wounded. Awareness of one's vulnerability can be both a blessing and a curse.

Support and feedback

Considering vulnerability, the wounded healer archetype can be a helpful metaphor for palliative care practice. The wounded healer is an ancient symbol that dates back to Greek mythology. More recently, the wounded healer archetype was popularized by Carl Jung, who posited that only the wounded physician can heal. Jung believed that the healer actually took over the suffering of the patient in the same way that combining two chemical substances creates a changed agent representing both substances.

Applying the wounded healer archetype to nursing practice, we may find ourselves in situations where we literally take on the feelings of our patients, and perhaps of their family members. This assumption of feelings can be a painful process and, while reflection can help in recognizing these dynamics, reflection alone is not enough.

It's essential for nurses working in these highly charged situations to get support and clinical consultation from trusted others. Clinical consultation may be provided by an individual or a group; regardless of the source, however, a prerequisite to helpful clinical consultation is your ability to trust in that person or group. Clinical consultation can serve multiple purposes; the two that will be highlighted here include validating affect and enhancing insight. (See *Validating affect and enhancing insight.*)

Reflection is typically triggered when something goes wrong. Otherwise, our actions are often on automatic pilot. But, when a glitch or a problem happens, we're called to the moment. We may ask, "What happened?" and consider the situation in more detail. If you use reflection alone, however, your own "truth" may be endlessly reinforced and your may not see things from another perspective.

Of course, you may not be ready to hear what you could do differently to alter the outcome of a situation. Certainly, if you're feeling sad and distressed, it's important to have your emotions validated. However, remaining open to considering alternative views will let you keep your perspective open and minimizes the chance that you'll experience burnout.

Likewise, if you're providing clinical consultation, ask: "Do you want support or do you want feedback?" Most people choose both—but support first. Asking that question encourages the other person to consider what she needs at that particular time. It also reinforces the notion that these are two different but complementary actions.

Also, consider that the wounded healer motif is different from the walking wounded motif. The wounded healer recognizes her vulnerability, while the walking wounded live with trauma without understanding its impact.

Every nurse brings a personal history to practice. Your personal history includes your previous experiences and your understanding of their meaning. (See *How to comfort a coworker*, page 284.) Working closely with dying people may propel you to experience your own vulnerability while also becoming more open to the experiences of others. This openness may lead to transformative moments that heighten your appreciation of life.

The helping relationship

Caregivers, especially female caregivers, have a tendency to attend to the feelings of others more than to their own feelings and needs. Focusing on interactions and the importance of relationships is a form of altruism that can be profoundly important in shaping our planet in positive ways. However, excessive self-sacrifice can leave one feeling angry, tired, even bitter.

It's essential that, as caregivers, we attend to our own needs as well as the needs of others. A first step in doing this is exploring our reasons for self-sacrifice. Offering the self should be a choice rather than an obligation. When one offers self out of choice, the self is enlarged rather than diminished.

Healthy self-sacrifice involves a balance on several levels. We balance taking care of others with taking care of ourselves. We balance autonomy with dependence. We balance our energy and our own needs. Healthy self-sacrifice emphasizes self-respect and a commitment to care of the self. Yet, in our culture we have little language that even describes how care for self and care for others should complement each other. We might learn from Eastern culture and belief systems such as Buddhism, which recognize the idea of intricate interdependence. Each of us is embedded in a living matrix that challenges the very notion of a dualism between autonomy and dependence.

Lack of self-care has historically been a problem in nursing; nursing education and practice may too often reinforce what Gordon calls the *virtue*

EXPERT INSIGHTS

How to comfort a coworker

I work with a nurse whose 16-year-old daughter died of leukemia about 7 months ago. She speaks to us about Sharon often and some-times even cries a bit. The other day I heard her conversing with a pa-tient who has the same oncologist Sharon had. They spent about 30 minutes talking and crying. Is this behavior appropriate? Do you think she should transfer out of the oncology unit for a while? — H.R., British Columbia

Let me tell you about Brenda. (She said I could.) Brenda is a great on-cology nurse, warm, funny, and caring. Her daughter Kim died of gas-tric cancer at age 21 — at home, in Brenda's arms.

Kim had been admitted many times on the oncology floor where Brenda works. During those hospitalizations, Brenda would take time off from work so she could stay with her daughter day and night. As Kim grew more ill, the staff nurses, who loved Brenda and her daugh-ter, had some emotionally difficult days caring for Kim, knowing she was running out of time.

When Brenda returned to work on the oncology floor after Kim's death, she was welcomed by a fantastic gang of nurses, mothers and fathers all. She's had good days and bad, but she carries on and con-tinues to give excellent care to her cancer patients. She speaks about Kim to them and shares special hope-filled books that have helped many patients and families during treatments and the terminal phase.

Some days I'll find her staring at a picture she carries of Kim, tears in her eyes. But if I try to give her a hug, she shoos me away saying, "Don't get me started, Joy. I don't want to cry."

I don't find any of this behavior inappropriate. If Brenda can't find compassion and understanding from her nurse-peers, we'd all be in trouble. I see no difference between comforting a patient who's mourning the potential loss of life and comforting a coworker mourn-ing the loss of a beloved daughter. If not here and now, then where and when?

— JOY UFEMA, RN, MS

script. The virtue script emphasizes self-sacrifice, altruism, and feeling con-tent that these virtues offer their own rewards. These messages contribute what remains as a caring dilemma in nursing, the perceived idea that nurs-es must care even when caring isn't valued by Western society.

> ## Qualities of healthy caregivers
>
> - **Purposeful use of self** — consciously and authentically using self as a therapeutic agent
> - **Lack of ego involvement** — recognizing self as part of but not central to the processes that another person is experiencing
> - **Empowerment though the use of resources** — keeping informed about appropriate resources and using these for care of self as well as care of patients
> - **Transcendence** — embracing the spiritual side of life
> - **Aesthetics** — appreciating the beauty of caregiving done from the heart
> - **Support** — using support and guidance for the work of caregiving

The helping relationship involves a person giving help, a person receiving help, and the value of the help itself. In palliative care nursing, choosing the right kind of help is essential. That involves not only knowing what is appropriate at one point for our patients and their families, but also being aware of what is needed for ourselves.

Traditionally, many of us have been socialized to be emotionally separate from our work, thus avoiding emotional upheavals. Although keeping emotionally distant may help us avoid getting involved, most of us come into this work to become involved and invested in the care of others. Devaluing care, or limiting our investment in care, separates us from the emotional satisfaction that comes from doing meaningful work.

There are road maps for identifying healthy aspects of caring. Self-awareness has already been addressed as an essential quality for healthy caregiving. In addition, other qualities are needed for healthy caregiving. (See *Qualities of healthy caregivers*.)

Level of expertise

Nurses develop skill along a beginner-to-expert trajectory. The job of the beginner is to master the multiple tasks required in nursing practice. As you grow in experience and expertise, you can participate in more of what makes excellent caregiving fulfilling and aesthetically pleasing. It's essential that experienced nurses are aware of this trajectory so as to be kind to nurses new to the palliative care field. Even nurses with several years of experience in other practice settings will be advanced beginners again when moving into a new practice area. Allowing the advanced beginner time to learn new clinical skills and supporting the learner along the way are methods of facilitating successful integration into palliative care.

Recognizing the trajectory involved in developing expertise may reduce the new nurse's feelings of role stress. Role stress has been described as the difference between a person's perceptions of a particular role and her achievement within that role. New nurses, especially, are at risk for role stress when their actual job performance doesn't match the expectations they have of what their performance should be. Role stress may also be worsened when dealing with "difficult" patients, families, and colleagues.

Dealing with difficulty

What makes a patient difficult? Each of us can probably recall a situation where a patient with whom we worked was a special source of discomfort for us. Whether we experienced anger, frustration, sadness, anxiety, or even fear, there was something about the interaction that created a problem for us. (See *Joshua and Candice*.) In a situation like Joshua's, you might have felt negative even before you'd met the patient. Often, this preliminary negative affect carries through, and you might find good reason to be even more negative toward the patient at the end of the shift.

Who's difficult?

The phenomenon of perceptual vigilance causes your attention to be drawn toward certain behaviors. Subsequently, if you believe that there will be a problem, you'll tend to find supporting evidence to confirm your belief. But, are people really difficult, or is it our response that creates difficulty for us?

When we label another person difficult, it's because we're looking at that person's behaviors rather than looking with them at the cause of the behaviors. The *looking at* process is one that we use when doing an assessment. We observe subtleties in breathing, skin color, and edema. During the mental status exam, we assess for affect (external manifestation of mood), thought process, and judgment. The looking at process enables us to recognize a rapidly deteriorating situation and to intervene before the situation becomes even worse. Looking at is an essential part of nursing practice.

Just as looking at is valuable, so too, is *looking with.* Looking with the patient has an important role to play in palliative care practice. Looking with involves considering what it might be like to be that other person. Looking with allows you to cultivate empathy for the other. Generally, the responses of others are understandable if you know what the other's point of view is. This knowledge involves paying attention to context, including the patient's history and his unique way of viewing the world. Let's return to the case example and consider how the patient may be feeling.

Candice's symptoms are becoming more severe. The things she previously used to cope — minimizing and denying — are no longer working

Joshua and Candice

Joshua Knight came onto his shift feeling good about the night ahead. He'd enjoyed a brisk run before work and had even found time to pack a dinner for his late-night shift. When he got to report, however, his mood changed. He was scheduled to work with Candice Taylor, a patient who was renowned for being difficult and demanding. Making matters worse, her daughter was coming to visit from out of town and planned to stay the night. Joshua groaned. Although he had never cared for Candice, her reputation was well known. "Why me?," he thought, "What did I do to deserve this?"

The patient

Candice Taylor was having yet another really bad afternoon. Her pain always got worse as the day wore on, which only reminded her how sick she was. She tried hard to forget about the sickness, but her body wasn't letting her. It was getting tougher to breathe, and she didn't have the strength to take care of herself the way she wanted to. And she felt so lonely and scared. Sometimes when others were in the room, she felt less afraid. She couldn't say why, just that she didn't feel as alone. But she knew the nurses didn't like her. And she was so thirsty again; that water just didn't taste right. She pressed the call bell again. The least she could get was some cold water!

The family

Maggie Taylor was distressed to see the amount of weight her mother had lost. She was furious at her mother for not calling sooner. What was her mom thinking?! Well, whatever she was thinking, Maggie figured it had something to do with her mom being on this unit. These nurses must not be feeding her enough. It's a good thing she'd come to take care of her mom. And she didn't want to hear any more of this doom and gloom the nurses were saying. That had to be making her mom feel even worse. How could somebody feel better when people were talking about dying and asking about living wills? She was going to tell the nurses to not give her mom any more bad news.

The crisis

Maggie cornered Joshua at the nursing station. "I don't like what's happening to my mom!" were her first words, said in anger. "I don't want you folks talking about dying. It's only making her feel worse. And I don't think a man should even be nursing her." Joshua worked to not respond in kind to Maggie's anger. In "looking with" her, he recognized that she was overwhelmed with her mom's deteriorating state. Rather than taking Maggie's comments personally, Joshua tried to process some of what Maggie might be feeling.

(continued)

Joshua and Candice *(continued)*

Joshua: "It must be tough to see your mom lose so much weight."
Maggie: "If you were feeding her better, she wouldn't be so skinny."
Joshua: "Her appetite seems to be changing. She's not so hungry these days. (silence) Is there any special food you think she might have an appetite for?" (silence)
Maggie: "I tried to get her to drink a chocolate milkshake. That's her favorite. But she won't have any of it."

---

well. As Candice's coping mechanisms fail to control her anxiety, she shows her feelings in other ways. She's frustrated because she's losing her ability to function. So, like many patients, she moves to control the things around her that she can control. Demanding cold water, which may be seen by the nurse as an irritating minor request, becomes Candice's way of taking some control over her experiences and of not feeling so alone.

The nurse who works to have insight into the patient's feelings and recognizes controlling behaviors as an attempt to get a handle on things that are beyond the patient's control will be better able to empathize with the patient. This empathy is essential because the patient is likely to feel less alone and abandoned. Unfortunately, what often occurs in these situations is that the nurse becomes more frustrated and tends to avoid the patient. This avoidance triggers the patient's fears and is likely to heighten the behavior.

Triangulation

The experienced nurse is skilled at both looking at and looking with, while also being aware that she brings self to interaction. So, what the nurse considers to be difficult may have more to do with the nurse than with the patient. Often, the patients who are most difficult for us are those who tap into some of our own issues. This recognition can be an important step in dealing more effectively with the patient as well as with our own feelings. Making matters more complex, of course, is that interactions hardly ever occur in isolation. Joshua is influenced by his colleagues and other members of the palliative care team. Candice is affected by her family members and may worry more about them than she does about herself. And once another person is added to a two-person system, there's the potential for triangulation. In triangulation, one person is drawn into a conflict between two other people, often to relieve some of the anxiety between the two people. So, how might this look in the situation with Joshua and Candice?

When looking with Maggie, it's easy to understand how she might be feeling. Her concern about the "doom and gloom" may be related to her fears that open discussion about the possibility of her mom dying would only lead to a loss of hope. We can also imagine how this kind of "protection" would begin to place the nurse in a bad position. Maggie's desire to protect her mom can put the nurse in the triangulated position between mom and daughter. If Joshua keeps an open conversation going, allowing Candice the space to talk about her fears for the future, Maggie is likely to be upset. Yet, if Joshua doesn't allow this open communication, he's less of an advocate for his patient.

Before addressing ways of dealing with the triangulated position, it's important to acknowledge the common and difficult situation in which family members disagree with each other or with the patient. What's your obligation for advocacy and support when there's a conflict between the needs of the patient and the needs of the family—all of whom are included in the unit of care? This ethical dilemma is one of the difficulties faced by nurses working in palliative care and a source of significant job-related anxiety and stress.

Consider the stress

Families face important challenges when dealing with the illness of a loved one. For example, a family dealing with a loved one who has Alzheimer's disease is faced with different challenges than a family trying to cope with cystic fibrosis in a child. A family dealing with relapsing-remitting multiple sclerosis faces different issues than those of a family dealing with amyotrophic lateral sclerosis. Recognizing that each family experiences unique stressors in dealing with the illness of a loved one, the astute nurse works to support the family's attempts at making sense of a difficult situation.

If you find yourself in a triangulated position, getting individual or group consultation can be helpful. A more intensive team approach to process the altered family dynamics may be needed. Preventing triangulation is the best strategy; this means refusing to take sides in a disagreement. You can recognize and validate each member's feelings, but avoid getting immersed in choosing one side over the other.

In the sample case crisis, Joshua continues to focus on Maggie's distress rather than reacting to her anger. He notes that Candice is "changing" and that these changes involve her appetite. Yet, understanding how distressing it is for family members to watch a loved one stop eating and become cachectic, Joshua does not openly confront Maggie's complaints. Nor does he try to educate Maggie on the appetite loss that is a normal part of the dying process; Joshua intuits that Maggie isn't ready for this type of information. The important point is that Joshua mentions that Candice is changing; in addition, Joshua gives Maggie some control by asking her what foods her mother might be interested in eating. Maggie acknowledges that her mom doesn't seem interested in even her favorite food, and the conversation has moved from adversarial to more collaborative.

Techniques to help families cope

■ Communicate effectively, and pace yourself to the family's communication pattern.
■ Provide skilled nursing care to control the patient's symptoms.
■ Allow family members to be present, and welcome their presence.
■ Coach family members on how they might participate in their loved one's care.

Of course, each family is different, and a good outcome doesn't always occur. In dealing with families, it's helpful to consider the amount of stress family members are facing during the times when they're feeling especially vulnerable. Recall that the term vulnerable means capable of being wounded. Also, consider that people experiencing severe stress tend to use the extremes of their coping mechanisms. A family member who copes by withdrawing during stressful times may isolate himself. A family member who copes by taking charge may become excessively controlling. (See *Techniques to help families cope.*)

Communication difficulties may also occur as a result of the family caregiver being displaced by the professional caregiver. It's essential to recognize that the family caregiver is likely an expert on the care of the patient. Considering the caregiver's point of view can help you incorporate caregivers into the ongoing plan of care. Information and support can then be provided in an individual manner rather than having a "one size fits all" model of dealing with primary caregivers. By "looking with" the patient and family, you're in a position to share knowledge with the family caregiver as well as to learn valuable lessons from that caregiver.

One recent study found that effective communication was one of the keys that physicians recognized as helpful in facilitating a good death. Conversely, communication marked by misunderstandings and conflict was related to a bad death. Yet, despite the recognized importance of good communication, many nurses still don't have the education they need to provide support for relatives when a patient is dying.

Although many communication difficulties with patients and family members may be resolved with effective nursing and team interventions, this isn't meant to condone abusive or hostile behavior. Violence in the workplace, including bullying and verbal abuse, are recognized as factors that influence recruitment and retention of nurses. If you're in a situation where you feel threatened—emotionally or physically—make use of the support available to you, ranging from clinical consultation to security or even police involvement.

Institutional influence

Institutional factors may significantly contribute to feelings of stress for the palliative care nurse. Completing burdensome paperwork and attending to numerous regulations may consume hours of time with little obvious reward. The setting itself may cause stress by being understaffed, mandating overtime hours, and forcing staff to use vacation time when the census is low. In a study on spirituality in nursing, nurses recognized system constraints that made delivering holistic care more difficult. (See *Hindrances to holistic care*.) Nurses who worked in hospice settings described receiving the most support for the spiritual dimension of their practice; nurses working in home-based settings also felt they had some time to devote to holistic nursing practice. However, nurses working in hospital settings experienced many limitations in delivering holistic nursing care.

Another salient issue in considering workload factors that contribute to stress for palliative care nurses is the nursing shortage. As the nursing workforce ages and patient care becomes ever more complex, nurses are required to care for sicker patients with less available support. These days, nearly three-fourths of nurses have a major concern about the acute and chronic effects of stress and overwork.

Staff conflicts

We all face numerous stressors in and out of the work setting. What's more, many palliative care nurses work in a culture that supports not making a fuss, speaking in a sympathetic voice even when angry, and putting the other person first, even when the other is taking advantage. Given this culture, some problems that are pervasive in many nursing settings include unwill-

---

Hindrances to holistic care

- **Inadequate time** — not enough quality time to spend with patients and family members
- **Rigid settings** — working in constricted models where technology is valued over touch
- **Lack of knowledge** — insufficient preparation for working with patients and families receiving end-of-life care
- **Lack of support** — not feeling comfortable talking with peers about beliefs or getting support from colleagues

ingness to openly confront, resentment because of self-sacrifice, and difficulty saying no.

Confrontation

Although many view it as negative, the term *confrontation* is defined as standing or meeting face to face. Confrontation involves dealing directly with our concerns. Many nurses feel uncomfortable with confrontation because they may have been socialized to believe that anger is bad and ultimately destructive. However, in healthy confrontation, people tell their own "truth" and remain open to the experiences of others. Confrontation involves "I" messages, taking responsibility for one's own feelings, and speaking in a clear manner without attacking the other. It also may be helpful to clearly describe a positive outcome to the confrontation. (See *Sharon and Tom.*)

Of course, we don't always get what we want when we ask for it; however, the first step in becoming more assertive is asking clearly and specifically for what we want. Notice that in the second example, Sharon was not openly angry; she spoke with Tom in a quiet place when they both had a bit of time available. She used "I" language and was clear about what she wanted. Even if Sharon didn't get a favorable response, she could walk away knowing that she had told her truth and done so clearly.

Resentment

Nurses are exposed to many messages that reinforce the virtue of taking care of other people. Sometimes (perhaps often) we neglect our own needs in the process, which can lead to resentment.

It's been said that we can't truly care for others if we can't care for ourselves. As a metaphor for this notion, consider the instructions given on an airplane. If the oxygen masks are released, passengers are instructed to put on their own masks before assisting others. The point, of course, is that oxygen deprivation doesn't increase alertness or the ability to help others.

It can be helpful to keep a barometer of self-sacrifice. Checking in to see what you're doing for others and balancing it with what you're doing for yourself can improve your physical, emotional, and spiritual health. And because behaviors may change on a day-to-day, perhaps even an hour-to-hour, basis, this is an area where frequent checking-in is especially helpful.

Learning to say "no"

Many of us slip into automatic pilot when asked to do yet another thing. We've missed the lesson that "no is a full sentence." Perhaps past experiences, including messages that were cultivated in your family of origin, have supported the idea that you need to do what others want you to do without considering your own needs. Here's another road to resentment; eventually, doing too much can push you into burnout and emotional exhaustion.

Sharon and Tom

Sharon Jones had had just about enough. Thomas Mass was, once again, asking her to cover his patients while he went to lunch. The problem was, Tom never reciprocated when Sharon wanted to go to lunch. Sharon decided she wasn't going to take it anymore. Here are two options she could use to confront Tom.

Option 1

Sharon approached Tom in the hallway, backing him against the wall. "You're always dumping on other people and I'm sick of it. Start pulling your weight around here," Sharon said loudly, and then walked away to cool off.

Option 2

During a slow period on the unit, Sharon sat down next to Tom as he was writing his notes. "Tom, I want to talk with you about something that has been bothering me. I usually cover your patients when you go to lunch, but when I ask you to do the same for me, you never seem willing." (silence) "I don't mind covering for you, but I'd like you to cover for me too."

"Really, I hadn't even thought of that. I'll pay more attention to it in the future," Tom replied, and then added, "Have you been to lunch yet? I have some time now."

The right way

In Option 1, Sharon approached Tom when she was feeling angry; she cornered him in a public place and verbally attacked him. This is exactly the wrong way to handle a confrontation.

Option 2 offers a better way. Using this approach, the story might even start differently, something like this: Sharon Jones had had just about enough. She decided to approach Tom to discuss her concerns.

Value of the team

One of the stress-protective factors mentioned in much of the literature on palliative care is the importance of the palliative care team. Yet, the interdisciplinary team may worsen stress in some situations, such as a lack of institutional support for training and resources. Education on communication skills for dealing with patients, family, and each other is essential to alleviating this source of stress.

Nurses new to palliative care are especially at risk for developing a medical model of care that emphasizes tasks and physical interventions. It's up to the palliative care team, and ultimately to the institution, to cultivate behaviors that include all aspects of the palliative care philosophy.

The interdisciplinary team is one of the hallmarks of hospice care. For nurses who work in hospice settings, the interdisciplinary team is often a source of support. However, when team roles aren't clearly defined, collaboration becomes difficult. In addition, the emphasis on technical skills and the expectation that team members are competent at these skills may cause tension in the palliative care team.

Given the importance of working together in a cohesive manner, it's essential that members of the interdisciplinary team treat each other with respect. Yet, there's some evidence that verbal abuse received by nurses in the work setting is more common from nurse colleagues than from any other source. Anger, judgment, criticism, and condescension can be common forms of verbal abuse encountered by nurses in the work setting. Some nurses can use direct communication to clear up misunderstandings and difficulties. Others are more passive, more silent—and more likely to avoid work (by calling in sick) and experience low job satisfaction.

Verbal abuse is an institutional problem; the culture of institutions either silently condones or openly rejects verbal abuse and bullying. Institutions are likely to be more effective at recruiting and retaining nurses when there's a zero-tolerance policy for abuse or bullying.

The burnout cycle

Burnout has been discussed extensively in the literature. (Some sources consider *compassion fatigue* a more helpful term than burnout.) Researchers have reported several interesting findings, including these:

■ Certain personality characteristics may make you more vulnerable to burnout, including being overly conscientious, perfectionistic, and self-giving.

■ Burnout involves emotional exhaustion, depersonalization of patients, and a low sense of personal accomplishment. (See *Common experiences in burnout.*)

■ Burnout may be related to the mixed recognition of palliative care work. Palliative care nurses are often praised, as their work is believed to be distasteful, but the actual clinical skills that drive this work are hidden, and thus devalued. Especially when framed as "women's work," the high levels of skills that are cultivated by excellent clinicians are easily disregarded.

■ Emotional exhaustion and depersonalization make nurses more likely to want to leave palliative care work.

■ Nurses with children tend to have lower depersonalization scores, which suggests that having children may increase job satisfaction.

■ Male nurses tend to report a lower sense of personal accomplishment than female nurses, putting them at higher risk of burnout.

■ Taking short breaks from work to deal with stress is one concrete way that some nurses improve their sense of personal accomplishment.

Common experiences in burnout

■ **High expectations.** You set yourself up to sacrifice your needs for the needs of your patients, which is self-destructive behavior.

■ **Intensity.** You become overly conscientious and may start to believe that you alone can solve a problem or help with a particular situation. You may find yourself reluctant to delegate and ask for help.

■ **Subtle deprivations.** You overlook your own needs and become consumed by your work.

■ **Altered coping mechanisms.** Your coping mechanisms become less healthy. You may be more irritable and less tolerant, and your sleep may be troubled.

■ **Dismissal of needs.** You grow out of touch with your body and your needs. You may develop symptoms of physical, psychological, or spiritual distress. And you may become frustrated by the amount of time you're spending on yourself if you do seek health care services.

■ **Distorted values.** You become excessively centered on the present, and doing so becomes the essential part of living.

■ **Denial.** Your perspective becomes severely impaired. Your thinking and attitudes may become rigid and inflexible. Tolerance declines, and you anger quickly over small things.

■ **Disengagement.** You become further separated from the outside world, and you may have a sense of hopelessness. You may avoid people, preferring to spend time alone or in isolating activities.

■ **Anhedonia.** You lose pleasure in life. What was once joyful is now an obligation. You have a sense of hollowness and emptiness.

■ **Observable behavior changes.** Friends and significant others notice that you've changed. You have less appreciation for the perspective of others. You may become irritated with what you view as interference and distance yourself from those who could support you.

■ **Depersonalization.** You feel separated from the world and possibly removed from reality, as though you're watching yourself from outside of your body.

■ **Emptiness.** You may feel hollow, drained, or depleted and may be more likely to turn to drugs, alcohol, or other excesses such as eating, shopping, or sex.

■ **Depression.** You feel a sustained state of sadness, lack of joy, despair, altered eating and sleeping, and possible thoughts of suicide.

■ **Burnout exhaustion.** In this crisis of total exhaustion, you feel completely depleted, emotionally, physically, and spiritually.

■ **Physical symptoms.** You may have chronic fatigue, headaches, back pain, GI problems, sleep disturbances, muscle tension, lingering illness, or vulnerability to illness.

Fighting burnout

■ Enhance commitment by reworking the situation internally, considering what you might do the next time a similar event occurs, such as expressing yourself directly to the other person involved in a conflict.
■ Increase control by seeking more information about the situation, reducing stress through activities such as physical exercise, changing the physical environment in some way, and searching for the spiritual meaning of a disturbing experience.
■ Build challenge by using interpersonal skills, expanding your perspective of a particular situation, and cultivating an intellectual attitude grounded in rationality.
■ Teach stress education and stress management in the workplace.
■ Use team-building strategies.
■ Work to balance priorities.
■ Enhance social support through engaging in social activities and peer support.
■ Allow for flexibility in work hours.
■ Have protocols in place to deal with violence.
■ Create opportunities for timely feedback.
■ Support autonomy of nursing practice.
■ Support further study and education.

It isn't clear whether nurses who work in palliative care are more or less likely than nurses working in other settings to experience high levels of stress and burnout. Certainly, ongoing contact with dying people can be intensely emotional and may evoke significant emotional turmoil. Watching family members suffer through the death of their loved one also may take a toll on nurses' well-being.

Burnout can have devastating consequences. Although change may occur at any point in the burnout cycle, intervening earlier rather than later is preferable. If you're looking at yourself and considering where you might fit on the burnout cycle, consider whether or not you still have perspective. Does your sense of humor seem to have disappeared? Are you taking life too seriously? Are you being too hard on yourself and others around you? If so, you have the opportunity to change your path and to cultivate healthier patterns of coping.

Preventing burnout

In addition to a zero-tolerance policy for verbal abuse and bullying, other strategies seem to work especially well in building a stress-resilient workplace. (See *Fighting burnout.*) These may focus on improving three components of psychological hardiness: commitment, control, and challenge.

■ Commitment is a sense of purpose and meaning experienced through active participation in life events.

■ Control is the belief that one's actions may influence life events.

■ Challenge is the recognition that change rather than stability is the norm in life.

Other strategies may work as well, particularly education. Educational opportunities can revitalize and stimulate nurses working in palliative care. If you have an associate degree or diploma, you may want to consider returning to school for a baccalaureate degree. If you have a baccalaureate degree, you may want to consider moving into graduate studies for an advanced practice role.

If you aren't interested in pursuing more formal education, conferences and conventions offer a way to keep up with what's going on in the field and to network with colleagues who have similar interests.

If you're not already certified, you may want to consider certification in palliative care nursing or oncology nursing. The National Board for Certification of Hospice and Palliative Nurses can be accessed at www.nbchpn.org. Oncology Nursing Certification Corporation information can be obtained from www.oncc.org. Certification information for pain management nurses may be accessed through the American Nurses Credentialing Center at www.nursingworld.org/ancc/.

Joining a professional organization may be well worth the price; membership in professional organizations gives you a national or international voice in your practice. Professional organizations provide countless opportunities for networking and education.

Another source of education that shouldn't be overlooked is the Internet. A reasonable strategy is to choose one or two sites of special interest and to periodically visit these sites to see updates. Many Web sites, such as Medscape.com offer free e-mail updates in specialty areas.

A Web site affiliated with the American Association of Colleges of Nursing has a special site devoted to end-of-life care. It provides extensive information about the End-of-Life Nursing Education Consortium (EL-NEC), a group whose main interest is in expanding the breadth and depth of this discipline. You can access the site at www.aacn.nche.edu/ELNEC/.

Personal coping strategies

Three factors influence whether a stressful time becomes a crisis time: coping mechanisms, perception of the event, and social support. Coping mechanisms are, simply stated, the ways in which we typically handle stress. (See *Growing the self,* page 298.) These patterns may be healthy and promote stress resilience, or they may be unhealthy and cause more distress. Coping mechanisms can include the use of humor, exercise, spiritual

---

Growing the self

- There's no single truth. Choose to cultivate activities that make sense to you.
- Rather than pathologizing your behavior and feelings, look at discomfort as an opportunity for growth.
- If you're feeling stuck, take a risk by doing one thing differently.
- Use your support system to help you cope during tough times. If you don't have a strong support system that lets you be vulnerable, develop one.
- Take time to cultivate what needs to be cultivated in you. Self-compassion is a wonderful gift you can give yourself.

---

venues, meditation, and leisure. Humor keeps us from taking ourselves too seriously and can be cultivated by encouraging moments of joy in the workplace. When used judiciously and with good timing, humor can also assist us in our difficult encounters with others.

Exercise in the form of any kind of physical activity can release endorphins (the "feel-good hormones") and stimulate emotional catharsis. For those who aren't used to being in motion, beginning with breathing and stretching exercises can be a useful way to start.

When we explore our spirituality, we consider meaning-making. How do we understand ourselves and our relationship to others on the planet? For what purpose do we exist? What is the meaning of suffering? Exploring spirituality for some of us may include cultivating our religious beliefs. Others may find solace in pondering spirituality through the written word.

Meditation is the practice of naturally preventing noisy thoughts by relaxing the body and trying to keep the mind "blank." There are many different meditation techniques.

Leisure activities are important sources of stress relief. They help with coping, and they improve work performance. They also are connected to spirituality, facilitate meaningful connections with others, and promote balance and integration. Activities such as cooking, music, arts, gardening, and physical labor are good examples of leisure activities.

Healthy ways of coping involve finding a balance in ourselves and cultivating that balance. Some of us find this balance by turning inward; we tend to be reflective and quiet, perhaps turning to solitary activities such as reading or meditating to become recentered. Others of us practice turning outward, where we find comfort and joy in the presence of others.

Jim and Mark

Jim Hayden couldn't believe that he was stuck behind the slowest driver on the planet. Today of all days! He was already running late for an important interview and had to stop for gas because he forgot to do so yesterday. Now, he had some guy ahead of him going 37 miles an hour in a 45-mile-an-hour zone. Of all the luck! Jim could feel his blood pressure rise as he pressed ever closer to this idiot's back bumper. His anger continued to rise as he was forced to wait at yet another light.

Mark Hopkins was having a tough day himself. He had just left the hospital, where he had spent the night in the emergency department with his wife. She was finally admitted to a room this morning. Now, the doctors were telling him that her breast cancer had metastasized to her liver and bones. He couldn't believe it. What was he going to tell his three kids? He drove slowly on automatic pilot, not even paying attention to the car that was easing ever closer to his bumper.

Widening perception

Many theoretical schools suggest that your perception of an event is more important than the event itself in determining your response. One such theoretical model is cognitive behavioral therapy (CBT). It's helpful to recognize that, generally speaking, a person's words and actions aren't not specifically designed to generate anger in others. Rather, it's our understanding of those words and actions that translates into negative feelings. This is a premise of CBT. (See *Jim and Mark*.)

How would this situation be different if Jim, who was rushing to get to an interview, knew about Mark's dilemma? Probably, Jim would have been less angry. Perhaps he even would have felt compassion for Mark.

An important point here is that the more we understand the context of a situation, the better we're prepared to handle that situation. Knowing that even the most irritating actions of others usually aren't designed to make our lives miserable can be an important step in expanding our own perspective.

Several books are available that teach strategies for changing our cognitive distortions. The idea is to recognize our negative thoughts, pick out the distortion we're using, and revise our cognitive statement. We're relearning our ways of understanding what we're experiencing.

Sources of social support

- Interdisciplinary team
- Clinical consultant
- Colleagues
- Friends and family
- Spiritual advisor, pastor, priest, rabbi
- Professional organizations
- Online support groups

Dialectic behavior therapy (DBT) is another option for dealing with our perceptions. In this therapy, dialectics — two apparent opposites — are brought together. For example, there may be times when I am a hard worker and there may be times when I am not such a hard worker and would rather sit around. Recognizing that both these descriptors apply to me can challenge my black-and-white thinking.

Social support

The third factor that determines whether or not a person goes into crisis is social support. Social support includes those people we can count on to help us during difficult times. Whether it's emotional support, financial help, babysitting, making dinner, or a variety of other behaviors, social support can be stress buffering. That is, it can actually tone down our experience of a stressful event. In some situations, social support can fully alleviate a stressor. (See *Sources of social support.*)

Intervening in burnout

If one is actually experiencing burnout, the above-mentioned prevention strategies may also be very helpful. Recognition is the first step in intervening in the burnout cycle. Once you can identify that you're experiencing symptoms of burnout, you have an opportunity to change direction. The first change that may be helpful is to re-evaluate your goals and priorities. What's really important, and how has that changed over time? What do I need to do to emphasize what's important in my life? A question that may be helpful in this evaluative process is: "What do I want to bring into my life?" Exploring resources for tapping into healthy coping mechanisms, broadening perspective, and seeking social support are likely to be helpful.

While the intent of this chapter isn't to diagnose or suggest treatment, it's important to seek assistance if depression is interfering with your functioning at work or at home. Also, if you've been having ongoing problems with eating and sleeping and haven't been able to find pleasure in your usual activities, you may be in need of help. If you've decided that you're expe-

Mental health care providers

- Advanced practice nurses (Some may prescribe drugs.)
- Masters-level social workers
- Masters- and doctoral-level psychologists
- Psychiatrists (Most prescribe drugs.)
- Clergy with specialized training in counseling

riencing depression and your attempts at changing this condition haven't helped, it may be time to consult with a qualified specialist. (See *Mental health care providers*.)

In addition to these providers, who typically have skills in psychotherapy, primary care practitioners (including physicians, nurse practitioners, and physician assistants) are often willing to prescribe antidepressants for their patients.

When seeking therapy, consider insurance coverage as well as the style of the psychotherapist. It's often possible to speak to a therapist on the phone and briefly explore his style. Many therapists specialize in certain methods; consequently, it's appropriate to get a preliminary sense of whether the therapist would be a "good fit." If medications are needed and these go beyond the scope of a primary care practitioner, then a psychiatrist or an advanced practice mental health nurse with prescriptive privileges would be best.

In some situations, group therapy is more helpful than individual therapy. Group therapy may be less expensive. Also, in a group setting, you have an opportunity to get feedback from several others rather than only one (the therapist). Groups can be very powerful and offer many benefits. There usually is a screening process involved in group therapy, so that the participants can be reasonably sure that other group members (like themselves) have met with the therapist to determine appropriateness for the group.

Hospitalization is usually reserved for those who have neurovegetative depression, suicidal ideation, or mixed substance abuse and depression. However, for some people with more complicated depression, hospitalization can be an important turning point on the road to recovery.

Working in palliative care is both invigorating and exhausting; our work pushes us to experience our vulnerabilities and allows us the option of evolving to become more of who we are as individuals and as moral beings. Yet, this growth often comes with a price. Your ability to identify your stressors and find ways to cope with them will help you gain the most from this challenging, rewarding work.

Caregiver resources

American Medical Association Caregiver Self-Assessment Tool
www.ama-assn.org/ama/pub/category/5037.html

Centers for Medicare and Medicaid Services
Medicaid Hotline (800) 633-4227
www.medicare.gov

Department of Health and Human Services Eldercare Locator
A national directory of community services
(800) 677-1116
www.eldercare.gov

Family Caregiver Alliance
(415) 434-3388
www.caregiver.org

National Alliance for Caregiving
(301) 718-8444
www.caregiving.org

National Dissemination Center for Children with Disabilities
(800) 695-0285
www.nichcy.org

National Family Caregivers Association
(800) 896-3650
www.nfcacares.org
see also www.familycaregiving101.org

Selected references

American Nurses Association. *Nursing's policy statement: Pain management and control of distressing symptoms in dying patients.* Washington, DC: American Nurses Association (nursebooks.org), 2003.

Beck, A.T., Epstein, N., Brown, G., and Steer, R. An inventory for measuring clinical anxiety: Psychometric properties. *Journal of Consultation and Clinical Psychology,* 56:893–7, 1988.

Carter, B.S., and Levetown, M.L., eds. *Palliative care for infants, children, and adolescents: A practical handbook.* Baltimore, MD: The Johns Hopkins University Press, 2004.

Clements, P., et al. Cultural perspectives of death, grief and bereavement. *Journal of Psychosocial Nursing,* 41(7):19–26, 2003.

D'Arcy, Y. Assessing pain in patients who can't communicate. *Nursing 2004,* 112:27, 2004.

Doyle, D., et al. *Oxford textbook of palliative medicine,* 3rd ed. Oxford, NY: Oxford University Press, 2005.

Erickson, J., and Millar, S. Caring for patients while respecting their privacy: Renewing our commitment. *Online Journal of Issues in Nursing,* 10(2), May 31, 2005.

Fox, E., et al. Evaluation of prognostic criteria for determining hospice eligibility in patients with advanced lung, heart, or liver disease. *JAMA,* 282:1638–45, 1999.

Francke, A.L., and Willems, D.L. (2005). Terminal patients' awareness of impending death: The impact upon requesting adequate care. *Cancer Nursing,* 28(3): 241–7, May/June 2005.

Goodlin, S., et al. Consensus statement: Palliative and supportive care in advanced heart failure. *Journal of Cardiac Failure,* 10:200–9, 2004.

Gordon, S. *Nursing against the odds.* Ithaca, NY: Cornell University Press, 2005.

Herth, K. Abbreviated instrument to measure hope: Development and psychometric evaluation. *Journal of Advanced Nursing,* 17:1251–9, 1992.

Hodgson, N.A., et al. Being there: Contributions of the nurse, social worker, and chaplain during and after the death. *Generations,* 28(2):47–52, 2004.

Hospice and Palliative Nurses Association. *HPNA position statement. Evidence-based practice,* 2004; p. 1–4. Retrieved September 20, 2005, from http://www.hpna.org/pdf/Position_EvidenceBasedPractice.pdf.

Hospice and Palliative Nurses Association and American Nurses Association. *Scope and Standards of Hospice and Palliative Nursing Practice.* Silver Spring, MD: Author, 2002.

Kerridge, I., et al. Death, dying, and donation: Organ transplantation and the diagnosis of death. *Journal of Medical Ethics,* 28:89–94, 2002.

Kuebler, K.K., Davis, M.P., and Moore, C.D. *Palliative practices: An interdisciplinary approach.* St. Louis: Mosby, 2005.

Laskowski, C., and Pellicore, K. The wounded healer: Applications to palliative care practice. *American Journal of Hospice and Palliative Care,* 19(6):403–7, 2002.

Levi, B. Withdrawing nutrition and hydration from children: Legal, ethical, and professional issues. *Clinical Pediatrics,* 42:139–45, 2003.

McCabe, C. Nurse-patient communication: An exploration of the patient's experience. *Issues in Clinical Nursing,* 13:41–49, 2004.

Moller, D. W. *Life's end: Technocratic dying in an age of spiritual yearning.* Amityville, NY: Baywood Publishing Co., 2000.

Moss, A., et al. ESRD workgroup final report summary on end-of-life care: Recommendations to the field. *Nephrology Nursing Journal,* 30(1):58–63, 2003.

National Consensus Project for Quality Palliative Care. *Clinical Practice Guidelines for Quality Palliative Care,* 2004; p. 1–76. Retrieved September 20, 2005, from http://www.aahpm.org/bookstore/index.html

Payne, N. Occupational stressors and coping as determinants of burnout in female hospice nurses. *Journal of Advanced Nursing,* 33(3):396–405, 2001.

Payne, S., Seymour, J., and Ingleton, C. (eds.). *Palliative care nursing: Principles and evidence for practice.* New York: Open University Press, 2004.

Price, C.A. Resources for planning and end-of-life care for patients with kidney disease. *Nephrology Nursing Journal,* 30(6):649–64, 2003.

Rando, T.A. *How to go on living when someone you love dies.* New York: Bantam Dell Publishing Group, 1991.

Robinson, J., and Crawford, G. Identifying palliative care patients with symptoms of depression: An algorithm. *Palliative Medicine,* 19:275–87, 2005.

Schonwetter, R., et al. Predictors of six-month survival among patients with dementia: An evaluation of hospice Medicare guidelines. *American Journal of Hospice and Palliative Care,* 20(2):105–13, 2003.

Searight H.R., and Gafford, J. Cultural diversity at the end of life: Issues and guidelines for family physicians. *American Family Physician,* 71(3):515–22, 2005.

SUPPORT principle investigators. A controlled trial to improve care for seriously ill hospitalized patients. The study to understand prognoses and preferences for outcomes and risks of treatment. *JAMA,* 274(20):1591–8, 1995.

Virik, K., and Glare, P. Validation of the Palliative Performance Scale for inpatients admitted to a palliative care unit in Sydney, Australia. *Journal of Pain and Symptom Management,* 23:455–7, 2002.

Westlake, C., et al. Depression in patients with heart failure. *Journal of Cardiac Failure,* 11:30–5, 2005.

Worden, J.W. *Grief counseling and grief therapy,* 3rd ed. New York: Springer Publishing Company, 2002.

World Health Organization. *Palliative care: Symptom management and end-of-life care,* 2003; p. 1-52. Retrieved September 26, 2005, from http://ftp.who.int/htm/IMAI/Modules/IMAI_palliative.pdf

Wright, L. *Spirituality, suffering and illness: Ideas for healing.* Philadelphia: F.A. Davis, 2005.

Yarbro, C.H., et al. *Cancer nursing principles and practice.* Sudbury, MA: Jones and Bartlett Publishers, 2005.

Index

i refers to an illustration; t refers to a table.

i refers to an illustration; t refers to a table.

i refers to an illustration; t refers to a table.

---

i refers to an illustration; t refers to a table.

i refers to an illustration; t refers to a table.

---

i refers to an illustration; t refers to a table.

---

i refers to an illustration; t refers to a table.

3